The Information Governance Toolkit

Data protection, Caldicott, confidentiality

Tobias Keyser
Professional Executive Committee Member
Information Governance Lead
Central Liverpool PCT

and

Christine Dainty
Associate Director
Mersey Deanery

Radcliffe Publishing
Oxford • San Francisco

Radcliffe Publishing Ltd
18 Marcham Road
Abingdon
Oxon OX14 1AA
United Kingdom

www.radcliffe-oxford.com
Electronic catalogue and worldwide online ordering facility.

British Library Cataloguing in Publication Data

A catalogue record for this book is available from the British Library.

ISBN 1 85775 600 2

Typeset by Aarontype Ltd, Easton, Bristol
Printed and bound by TJ International Ltd, Padstow, Cornwall

Contents

Preface   vi
About the authors   ix
Acknowledgements   x
List of abbreviations   xii

Part One   1
Tobias Keyser

Chapter 1: Information governance   3
Caldicott Report   5
Caldicott Principles   8
Section 1:   Caldicott Guardian/Information Governance Lead   10
Section 2:   Staff code of conduct   12
Section 3:   Staff induction procedures   21
Section 4:   Confidentiality and security training needs   24
Section 5:   Communication with patients/information for patients 26
Section 6:   Staff contracts   33
Section 7:   Contracts placed with other organisations   35
Section 8:   Reviewing information flows   39
Section 9:   Information/data 'ownership'   45
Section 10: Safe-haven procedures   47
Section 11: Protocols to govern information sharing   55
Section 12: Security policy   57
Section 13: Security responsibilities   63
Section 14: Risk assessment and management   65
Section 15: Security incidents   69
Section 16: Security monitoring   73
Section 17: User responsibilities   76
Section 18: Access controls   78
Section 19: Information governance assessment   83
Section 20: Implementation strategy   91

Chapter 2: Data Protection Act 1998   95
The Data Protection Principles   95
Explanatory notes about the Data Protection Principles   96
Individuals' rights   102
CCTV and Commissioner's Code of Practice (section 51(3)(b) DPA 1998) 106

Chapter 3: Other important legislation and guidance   **117**
Common law duty of confidentiality   117
Human Rights Act 1998   117
Crime and Disorder Act 1998   118
Health and Social Care Act 2001, section 60   119
Freedom of Information Act 2000   120
Access to Health Records Act 1990   123
Computer Misuse Act 1990   123
Copyright, Designs and Patents Act 1988   123
Public Interest Disclosure Act 1998   124
Children's Act 1989   124

Part Two   **127**
Christine Dainty

Chapter 4: Applying Caldicott to general practice   **129**
Introduction   129
Information for patients   129
Staff conduct and patient confidentiality   131
Staff induction and training   132
Confidentiality agreements   134
Data ownership   136
Safe haven   138
Security monitoring   140
Physical threats   142
Software and computer viruses   144

Chapter 5: Practical aspects of confidentiality, Caldicott   **147**
         and access
Introduction   147
Retention of records   147
Quality of record keeping   149
Access to records   151
Patient consent to access medical information   153
Complaints procedure   154
Confidential waste   156
Electronic communications   158
Publication scheme   161
Significant event analysis   163
The new GP contract   165
Further information   168

Chapter 6: Practice policies   **171**
Introduction   171
Incorporation of policies into general practice   173
Essential components of a policy   174
Dissemination of policies   175
Monitoring the effectiveness of policies   175

Practice leaflet   177
Practice complaints policy   179
Office policy   182

Appendix   **187**

Further reading   **195**

Glossary   **197**

Index   **201**

Preface

Confidentiality in the relationship between patient and doctor/primary healthcare team (PHCT) is a cornerstone in the medical practice. Only when the patient is sure that their information is treated confidentially will they be able to seek help without fear that their rights on privacy, dignity and integrity are at risk. This means that the patient is not only sure that all information about them is treated confidentially but also that they are in control of what happens with that information. Although the highest possible standard of confidentiality should be required merely for its beneficial effect on all dealings with a patient, there is a legal obligation as well. The proper handling of patient information is a legal responsibility of PHCTs and NHS organisations.

The modernisation of the NHS, increasing its efficiency and effectiveness through developments and more extensive use of information management and technology (IM&T), improved the capacity to make information about patients more extensively, rapidly and widely available. Although this has clear benefits for the patient in giving healthcare professionals prompt and comprehensive understanding of the patient's medical and social situation, and providing seamless multi-agency and integrated care, it poses a significant dilemma. The increased 'availability' of patient data will make the protection of confidentiality and the safeguarding of data – especially against unauthorised or inappropriate access – more difficult.

The increasing computerisation and use of telecommunication pose another problem – the wide dissemination of patients' health information renders the concept of 'location' of such information meaningless, compared to the paper records which were solely under the control of the treating health professional.

A further 'problem' concerning the confidentiality of patient data is the essential requirement for the NHS to collect specific data which are not needed for the immediate or direct care/treatment of the patient but which are very important for the operational needs of the NHS, i.e. for the monitoring and securing of public health (e.g. sexually transmitted diseases [not HIV], *E coli* outbreaks), monitoring and securing standards of healthcare provision (e.g. clinical governance, audits, evaluation of treatments), administrative needs (e.g. accounting, management and planning of services, monitoring of performance), as well as other important NHS tasks such as teaching and research.

Information governance, embracing Caldicott and the Data Protection Act 1998, provides the framework within which the above issues are addressed. Caldicott and the Data Protection Act overlap and complement each other in the aim of securing patient confidentiality and transparent data usage. The Data Protection Act 1998 emphasises not only the transfer of patient information but also its collection, which has to be performed with great care. It builds on the initial Data Protection Act of 1984. The 'revised' Act takes into account the increasing use of computer databases to store patient information. This legislation extends and increases the responsibility on data controllers to handle such information within a legal framework and means that health professionals are legally obliged to complete, update and retain paper (i.e. 'manual') and computer records in a proper manner.

Caldicott and the 'new' Data Protection Act 1998 give patients more rights and those who handle confidential information more responsibilities, and will ultimately change the way in which health professionals handle confidential information. However, the need for change should not result in harming or providing a lower standard of care for the patient/client, unless the patient chooses not to share certain information necessary to provide a high standard of care.

In 1998, the Department of Health (DoH) published the 'Caldicott Audit Questionnaire' setting out the items by which organisational performance on confidentiality and security can be assessed against the standards set by the Caldicott Committee. This audit was carried out in 2000 on a cross-section of practices in Liverpool and showed that in these practices significant improvements in the set-up of information governance were needed.

As a result of these findings a *Manual for Primary Healthcare Teams* was developed for Central, North and South primary care trusts (PCTs) in Liverpool. Following its successful introduction frequent requests for copies were made from other PCTs and this has led to the writing of *The Information Governance Toolkit*. This *Toolkit* contains practical advice on, and solutions for, developing issues of information governance in PHCTs. It does not deal with the social, judicial, financial, medical and educational implications. Neither does it deal with shortcomings and conflicts between different pieces of legislation and guidelines. The practical aspects such as assistance, advice and solutions in developing issues of information governance were given priority, and theoretical questions are not discussed. The *Toolkit* has the following aims:

1 Increasing PHCTs' knowledge base on information governance.
2 Effective, efficient and rapid improvement in the standards of data protection and confidentiality and overall performance in information governance within PHCTs, despite financial and time constraints.
3 Providing assistance in documenting the appropriate handling of information governance by providing the necessary forms.
4 Providing clear and concise guidance and help for PHCTs in developing their own policies for staff by bringing the relevant legislation and publications together.

The *Toolkit* should also convince PHCTs that the great effort and expense needed for achieving the goals of information governance are worthwhile because they will gain greater patient trust, better patient care and help with NHS modernisation.

Readers are reminded to use the *Toolkit* in conjunction with the latest DoH guidelines and legislation on information governance.

We hope this *Toolkit* achieves its goals and provides the help it sets out to give. We welcome reader feedback and any suggestions for improvement.

Tobias Keyser MD, MRCGP, DRCOG, DFFP
Professional Executive Committee Member
Information Governance Lead
Central Liverpool PCT
August 2004

Email: tobias.keyser@centralliverpoolpct.nhs.uk

About the authors

Tobias Keyser MD, MRCGP, DRCOG, DFFP was born in 1963 in Marburg, Germany. He studied law at the University of Cologne between 1984 and 1986, before entering medical school at the same university. His medical studies took him to the Worksop Hospital, Nottinghamshire, in 1989, and in 1990 to Australia to the University of Melbourne and Toowoomba Base Hospital. He spent the final year of medical school at the University of Missouri, Columbia, USA. He began work in the NHS in 1993 at the Royal Liverpool University Hospital and in 1997 he received his medical doctorate (MD) from the University of Cologne. He has been a general practitioner in Everton, Liverpool, since 2000. During 2000–2001, he was Caldicott Lead of Merseylive Primary Care Group (PCG) in Liverpool, and since 2001 he has been a Professional Executive Committee Member of the Central Liverpool Primary Care Trust, for which he is also Information Governance Lead.

He is also the Honorary Secretary of the Mersey Faculty of the Royal College of General Practitioners and a GP trainer.

Christine Dainty BSc Hons, MBChB, MRCGP, Cert Med Ed is an associate director for Mersey Deanery. Her previous experience as a full-time GP, GP trainer and GP tutor has encompassed a wide range of educational activities for individuals and multidisciplinary groups. Her current remit in the Deanery is vocational training, supporting doctors during their hospital placements. She also works with local primary care trusts and is involved with First Contact Practitioner initiatives. She obtained her certificate in medical education from Stafford University in 2002. At present she is combining her general practitioner skills with a GPwSI role in emergency care at St Helens and Knowsley Trust.

Acknowledgements

TK. I would like to thank Dr Ed Gaynor (previously Chair of Merseylive PCG), Maria Cody (previously Community Service Manager, Merseylive PCG) and Dr Jeff Featherstone (previously Clinical Governance Lead, Merseylive PCG) for their helpful comments during the development of the *Caldicott Manual for Primary Health Care Teams* which formed the basis for Part One of this book.

CD. I would like to acknowledge my colleagues in the Mersey Deanery for all their support they have given me during this undertaking. I would also like to thank South Sefton PCT Medicines Management Team, for their contribution towards the prescribing audit tool.

TK

This book is dedicated to my wife Janet, son Alexander, and my parents Helmtraud and Peter Keyser for their love, help and support.

CD

To my daughter, Christina, with love.

List of abbreviations

BMA	British Medical Association
CCTA	Central Computer and Telecommunications Agency
CCTV	Closed circuit television
DoB	Date of birth
DoH	Department of Health
DPA	Data Protection Act 1998
FoI	Freedom of Information Act
GMC	General Medical Council
GMS	General Medical Services
HRA	Human Rights Act
IM&T	Informatviiiviiiviiiviiiviiiion management and technology
IT	Information technology
NHS	National Health Service
NICE	National Institute for Clinical Excellence
NSF	National Service Framework
PCG	Primary Care Group
PCO	Primary Care Organisation
PCT	Primary Care Trust
PHCT	Primary Healthcare Team
PIAG	Patient Information Advisory Group
PMS	Personal Medical Services
PRIMIS	Primary Care Information Service
RCGP	Royal College of General Practitioners
SEVA	Significant event audit

Part One

Tobias Keyser

Chapter 1

Information governance

In the face of new developments in information technology and rapid computerisation the NHS must do its best to ensure that patient information is processed fairly, respectfully, confidentially, and is secured from uncontrolled, unauthorised and inappropriate access. Being aware of these requirements the primary healthcare teams (PHCTs) are increasingly expected to work in close collaboration with the NHS and non-NHS organisations to provide seamless, effective and rapid care for its clients. In addition the NHS needs to balance potentially conflicting needs of patients' wishes to secure and keep their data confidential and its own needs for patient information to remain operational.

All these demands make the handling of information a very complex and difficult task, which has increasingly required regulation in order to satisfy all the mentioned requirements and ensure that the handling of information is legitimate, of a high standard and protects patient confidentiality. Information governance provides the guidance for everybody involved in these processes.

It does so by bringing together all existing guidance, regulations and legal and statutory requirements and provides a framework for the handling of information in a confidential and secure manner within appropriate ethical and quality standards in a modern health service.[1] It aims at giving the clients of the health service more choice and control over their personal information.

The foundation of the framework for information governance is provided by legislation as well as the NHS and professional body guidance. The main legislation and legal requirements are:

- the common law duty of confidentiality
- Data Protection Act 1998
- Human Rights Act 1998
- Freedom of Information Act 2000
- Computer Misuse Act 1990
- Access to Medical Reports Act 1988
- Access to Health Records Act 1990
- Crime and Disorder Act 1998
- Health and Social Care Act 2001
- Human Fertilisation and Embryology Act 1990
- Copyright, Designs and Patents Act 1988, Copyright Regulations 1992
- Electronic Communications Act 2000
- Public Interest Disclosure Act.

The main published guidance of the NHS and professional bodies are:

- the Caldicott Report 1997
- *Confidentiality: NHS Code of Practice*, DoH, version 3.0, 2003
- BS 7799-1:1999 *Information Security Management – Part 1: Code of practice for information security management*
- *Ensuring Security and Confidentiality in NHS Organisations, protecting the security of information in NHS organisations*, NHS Executive's Security and Data Protection Programme, IMG Ref No E5501
- *The Handbook of Information Security: information security in general practice*, published by the NHS Executive's Security and Data Protection Programme
- *For the Record*, HSC 1999/012
- *Preservation, Retention and Destruction of GP General Medical Services Records Relating to Patients*, HSC 1998/217
- PRIMIS data quality
- data accreditation
- controls assurance standards (IM&T and records management)

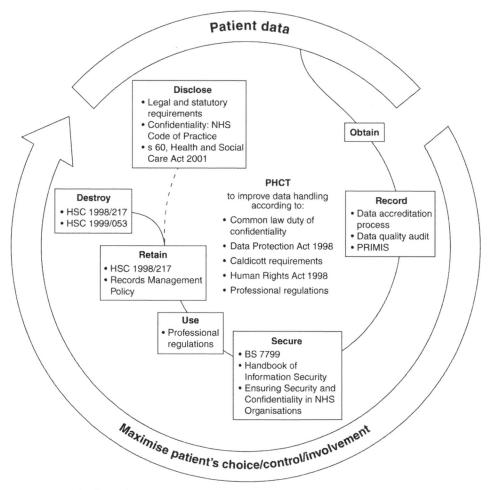

Figure 1.1 The flow of patient data with illustrating examples of regulations which shape this flow.

- NHS sexually transmitted disease regulations 2000
- GMC *Confidentiality: protecting and providing information.*

So, one main objective of information governance is to give guidance on the handling of patient data. Focusing on the needs of PHCTs Figure 1.1 illustrates the flow of patient data in its context with examples of regulations which shape this flow.

The flow of patient data in PHCTs as shown here starts with the obtaining of the data. They are then recorded and secured, and after their use are retained (for a specified period of time). The data might be disclosed and finally destroyed. These processes are regulated for example by the common law duty of confidentiality, the Data Protection Act 1998, Caldicott requirements, and others. Most of these processes have their own additional regulations (for example HSC 1998/217 and HSC 1999/053 for the destruction of personal data).

However, information governance should not just be seen to be dealing with personal information as its definition should be extended in order to take into account the Freedom of Information Act 2000, which obliges the health service (including the PHCTs) to provide information that facilitates operational transparency.

The most important components of information governance are the standards of the Data Protection Act 1998, dealt with in Chapter 2, and the Caldicott requirements following the Caldicott Report. The latter not only gives recommendations on the handling and transmission of patient data but also urges an educational and supervisory system to ensure its implementation.

Caldicott Report

The Caldicott Report was the result of the work of a committee, chaired by Dame Fiona Caldicott and published in December 1997. The Chief Medical Officer had established this committee to look at the transfer of patient-identifiable information between NHS organisations and with non-NHS organisations for purposes other than immediate treatment/care.[2,3] Thereby he had responded to previous publications of the Department of Health (DoH), *The Protection and Use of Patient Information*[4] (published in 1996, replaced in 2003 by the document *Confidentiality: NHS Code of Practice*)[5] and further work undertaken by a British Medical Association (BMA) Working Group about *Security in Clinical Information Systems* (published in 1996).[6]

The Caldicott Committee Report made 16 recommendations — some of which have been to some degree superseded by the new GMS (general medical services) contract — with a view to developing and implementing a new framework for handling patient information in the NHS:

- Recommendation 1
  Every transfer of patient information, including potential transfers, has to adhere to the six Caldicott Principles (which are outlined following these recommendations).
- Recommendation 2
  All NHS organisations are to establish a permanent programme for their employees to ensure that the highest standards of patient confidentiality and information security are achieved and a high level of awareness is continuously kept.

- Recommendation 3
  A network of Caldicott Guardians should be established. Every NHS organisation should nominate a senior member as a Guardian who will be in charge, facilitate and oversee the organisation's development to high standards of patient confidentiality and information security.
- Recommendation 4
  Guidance needs to be developed for all cases when patient-identifiable information may be used.
- Recommendation 5
  Protocols and systems need to be developed to safeguard the patient-identifiable information shared between NHS organisations and with non-NHS organisations.
- Recommendation 6
  The person in each organisation – most likely the Guardian – who is responsible for the monitoring of shared and transferred information needs to be clearly identified within and outside the organisation.
- Recommendation 7
  The committee suggests an accreditation system that certifies organisations with good procedures of safeguarding patients' confidentiality.
- Recommendations 8 and 13
  Wherever possible, and as soon as possible, the new NHS number should replace other patient-identifiable data. The use of data for patient identification other than the new NHS number has to be well justified.[7] A continuing effort should be made to increase the usage of the new NHS number where other means of patient identification – name, address, postcode, date of birth (DoB) – have not been used so far in primary care.
- Recommendation 9
  Protocols need to be developed specifying who and under which circumstances a person is authorised to have access to a patient's identity where a coded identifier (such as the new NHS number) is used.
- Recommendations 10, 11 and 14
  The Caldicott Committee urges the improvement of privacy-enhancing technology and its more extensive usage.[8,9] It also commends that anybody or any company involved in the supply or development of information systems for the NHS has ensured that the highest standard of privacy-enhancing technology has been incorporated, i.e. wherever possible privacy-enhancing technology should be used in the design of new IM&T systems, e.g. the electronic transfer of prescriptions.
- Recommendation 12
  Databases (existing and those to be developed) should be restructured, if practical, separating administrative (patient identifiers) from clinical information (such as conditions, treatments etc.), so the linking of administrative with clinical information will only happen under controlled and authorised circumstances.
- Recommendations 15 and 16
  Payments to GPs (general practitioners) should avoid systems requiring patient-identifiable information and new procedures for GP payment without the use of patient-identifiable information ought to be piloted.

Consultations on the Caldicott Committee Report emphasised that the protection and use of information — largely collected by health professionals from patients, in confidence, to support the delivery of care — was a part of the overall quality of care and was therefore an important component of clinical governance. The government is committed to the implementation of the recommendations of the *Caldicott Committee Report on the Review of Patient-identifiable Information*.[10] The *Report* therefore constitutes a major part of information governance.

In the following sections key terms and regulations of information governance are described and explained to facilitate their practical application in primary care, followed by chapters on data protection and other legislation and guidance.

Caldicott Principles

The Caldicott Principles[11] are guidelines as to what should be observed when information about patients needs to be passed on (either within or to anyone outside the practice). Any member of staff (clinical or non-clinical) passing on information about patients must abide by these rules.

1 *Justify the purpose(s).*
   Every proposed use or transfer of patient-identifiable information within or from your practice should be clearly defined, scrutinised and continual uses regularly reviewed.
2 *Do not use patient-identifiable information unless it is absolutely necessary.*
   Patient-identifiable information items (such as name, address, date of birth) should not be used unless there is no alternative.
3 *Use the minimum necessary patient-identifiable information.*
   When the use of patient-identifiable information is considered to be essential, each individual item of information should be justified with the aim of reducing identifiability.
4 *Access to patient-identifiable information should be on a strict need-to-know basis.*
   Only those individuals who need access to patient-identifiable information should have this access, and they should only have access to the information items they need to see.
5 *Everyone should be aware of his/her responsibilities.*
   Action should be taken so that clinical and non-clinical staff become aware of their responsibilities and obligations to respect patient confidentiality.
6 *Understand and comply with the law.*
   Every use of patient-identifiable information must be lawful. Someone in the practice should be responsible for ensuring that the practice complies with legal requirements.

© Crown copyright

References

1 NHS Information Authority. http://www.nhsia.nhs/infogov/pages/default. asp
2 DoH (1997) *The Caldicott Committee Report on the Review of Patient-identifiable Information*, December. http://www.hmso.gov.uk/confiden/app2.htm
3 Although the Caldicott Report initially applied to the NHS, its rules were introduced to social services in 2002. HSC 2002/003: LAC (2002)2, 31 January 2002.
4 DoH (1996) *The Protection and Use of Patient Information*, HSG(96)18/ LASSL(96)5.
5 DoH (2003) *Confidentiality: NHS Code of Practice*, version 3.0. http://www. doh.gov.uk/ipu/confiden
6 Dr Ross J Anderson (1996) *Security in Clinical Information Systems*, January. Consultation paper commissioned for the BMA Council by the BMA Information Technology Committee.

7   However, if the new NHS number cannot be validated at the time of entry, e.g. handwritten records, then additional items, such as sex or date of birth, may be used to minimise problems through transcription errors.

8   This is also a requirement of the Data Protection Act 1998. It is not feasible for an individual GP practice to develop its own IT (information technology) system capable of concealing patient-identifiable information but if these features are available they must be used on a need-to-know basis to maximise patients' privacy.

9   The NHS, DoH, BMA and the clinical professions have agreed that patient-identifiable information should be encrypted before being disclosed via any external network. *See* encryption and cryptography section of http://www. nhsia.nhs.uk/confidentiality/pages/standards.asp.

10   DoH (1998) *A First Class Service: consultation document.*

11   DoH (1997) *The Caldicott Committee Report,* p 17.

Section 1
Caldicott Guardian/Information Governance Lead

In the literature on handling of patient data there are several different titles for persons to whom the responsibilities for data protection, confidentiality and data security are assigned e.g. Caldicott Guardian,[1] Information Governance Lead, Caldicott lead, data protection lead, data protection officer, information security officer and so on. These job titles often lack clear distinctions of their specific roles as they have very similar responsibilities with significant overlaps. This section will not attempt to define these different roles but suggest – as a practical solution – what person specifications and job responsibilities are needed to improve and develop all aspects of data protection in primary care. If your PHCT already has a nominated person, it would be worthwhile if necessary to widen their remit rather than renaming their job and developing new structures. This book will use the term 'Caldicott Guardian' as it has been established since 1997 and (re-)define the person specifications and job responsibilities specific for the needs of a PHCT. However, whatever job title is chosen it is of the utmost importance that it should be very clear from within and outside the PHCT who is in charge of data protection, confidentiality and data security for your PHCT.

In a single-handed GP practice the GP will ultimately be responsible for data protection, confidentiality and data security, but in group practices one GP, e.g. the senior partner, should be nominated to take on these responsibilities. They may be delegated to another senior member of staff.

Person specifications:

- senior (preferably clinical) member of the PHCT team
- strong links to PHCT clinical governance lead, preferably the same person
- needs the respect and has the support from all senior members of staff and preferably the whole PHCT
- through his/her position in the PHCT must be able to initiate changes, develop policies, enforce adherence to policies
- takes on a strategic role
- can take influence on the commitment of resources
- is adequately trained
- is able to commit the necessary time to fulfil this role since key responsibilities should not be delegated.

Job responsibilities/description/role:

- keeping up to date via continuous and adequate training and keeping log of training received
- keeping up to date with changes of legislation
- networking with other PHCTs' and PCOs' (primary care organisations) Caldicott Guardians/Information Governance Leads to minimise duplication of effort, and improve on existing policies
- ensuring that effective procedures of communication with patients are in place
- risk management

- overseeing CCTV (closed circuit television) policies
- producing annual reports as a result of annual audits on data protection, confidentiality and information security
- developing annual improvement plans
- ensuring that all the practice's policies are in line with national guidance and have been approved by the PCO's Caldicott Guardian
- ensuring compliance with policies
- ensuring the implementation and enforcement of policies
- reviewing policies and monitoring their effectiveness
- facilitating the training of members of staff
- ensuring that the practice's data protection notification to the Office of the Information Commissioner is comprehensive (i.e. all databases that require registration are registered in accordance with the Act's requirement)
- keeping the registration up to date and reviewing regularly that the procedures for processing personal data are in place
- ensuring that disclosures of information are checked against the registrations
- ensuring that all members of staff are given access to confidential information on a need-to-know basis and keeping an up-to-date registration of IM&T users
- providing expert advice on issues of data protection and on disclosure of confidential information.

Reference

1   HSC 1999/012 outlines the person specification and role of the Guardian.

Section 2
Staff code of conduct

Every member of staff should comply with this code of conduct and be made aware of his/her responsibilities and that any breaches of this code could result in disciplinary action.[1–3] Everyone should receive a copy of this code of conduct and it should be reviewed on a regular basis. The following will outline the basic principles (you might like to print these principles from www.radcliffe-oxford. com/informationgov).

- All information from and about patients is to be treated confidentially, and their privacy, dignity and integrity has to be protected and respected at all times.[4]
- Every member of staff (practice or attached staff) has an obligation to safeguard the confidentiality of any personal information.[5]

  Although this is part of common law and may also be part of the professional code of conduct this should also be included in contracts of employment. Staff need to be aware that any breach of confidentiality could be a matter for disciplinary action and provides grounds for complaints against them.
- Everyone with access to patient-identifiable information (i.e. name/initials, address/postcodes, date of birth/death or any other dates, NHS number, NI (national insurance) number, ethnicity, job etc.) should be aware of his/her responsibilities, understand the law and comply with it.[6]

  The Data Protection Principles and Caldicott Principles define these responsibilities. Every member of staff should also comply with information technology security.
- Information about a patient should not be released without authorisation from the patient with an explicit consent or if explicitly permitted by the legislation.[7]

  In general, any personal information given or received in confidence for one purpose should only be used related to the purpose for which the information was collected and may not be used for a different purpose or passed to anyone else without the consent of the provider of the information. Special awareness is needed that consent is obtained if patient-identifiable information is used for purposes other than direct patient care.
- Patient-identifiable information should only be used if absolutely necessary and the purpose is justified.[8]
- Every member of staff should be aware of his/her responsibilities in safeguarding the integrity and availability of patient data.[9]
- Access to and distribution of personal information should be on a strict *need-to-know* basis.[10]

  Disclosures of identifiable information should be limited to the minimum necessary to accomplish the purpose of the disclosure.
- Individuals' wishes with regard to the 'handling' of their personal data should be respected as long as this is lawful.[4]

  If an individual wants information about them to be withheld from someone, or some agency, which might otherwise have received it, the individual's wishes should be respected unless there are exceptional circumstances. The individual needs to understand the consequences of such a request regarding his/her care.

**The following rules should be observed and form a part of the
responsibilities and duties of *every member* of staff in the practice
(you might like to print these rules from www.radcliffe-oxford.com/
informationgov).**

- The above principles apply to all patient information and confidential data (i.e. phone messages, word by mouth, computer or paper records, lab results, letters, photos/images/videos) in your working environment which includes the patient's relatives and carers, staff and colleagues from your PHCT or any other organisation.
- Do not give your password to another person and follow all the guidance on passwords (*see* Section 18, Access controls).
- Follow 'clear desk and clear screen' policy and other guidance in User responsibilities section (*see* Section 17).
- Follow the policy of log-on/log-off procedures (*see* Section 18, Access controls).
- Follow guidance on disclosure policy (end of this section).
- Do not discuss patient details within earshot of a third party.
- No patient records or details should be left in areas where an unauthorised person might gain unsupervised access to or be able to read any parts of the records.
- Records should be kept accurate and up to date.
- Be aware of and follow the code of practice for recorded images/CCTV.
- Patient-identifiable information should only be disposed via crosscut-shredding or incineration or a designated 'confidential' waste bag.
- Any breaches or potential breaches of confidentiality should be brought to the attention of your line manager and be logged (*see* Section 15, Security incidents).
- Understand and comply with the Data Protection Principles and the Caldicott Principles and security policy (*see* Section 12).
- Observe guidance produced by your professional or regulatory body.

Telephones

- Only give out information by telephone if you are sure that you are speaking to the right person.
- Your PHCT should develop a protocol to establish the type of information that may be disclosed over the telephone.
- Your PHCT should also develop safeguards to minimise the risk of disclosing information to the wrong person, e.g. procedures of identifying the patient, use of call-back procedures using published phone numbers. If there is any doubt about the person's identity on the phone, information should not be disclosed.

Email/Internet

- Regulations on email are identical to any other form of correspondence (Caldicott and Data Protection Principles apply) and can be legally binding or challenged. PHCT staff should ensure when using the Internet that they comply with their PCO's policies on Internet and emails.
- The Internet should only be used for non-confidential information exchange.

- The NHS Code of Connection regulates the connections to NHSnet. PHCT staff must adhere to the guidance on good practice developed by the NHS Information Authority. All connections wherever possible should be made through the NHSnet.[11]

Answering machines

- Messages left on answerphones should only be taken when the authorised person alone can hear them.
- Answerphones should be located in areas where only authorised persons have access to them and should be locked away when unattended.
- Any patient information received by answerphones should be treated with the same level of confidentiality as any other confidential information.
- The pre-recorded message should clearly state who will take the messages at a later stage, i.e. the doctor, senior receptionist/receptionist or the practice nurse.

Fax machines[12]

- The fax machine should be placed in a location (i.e. safe-haven, see Section 10, Safe-haven procedures) where only authorised persons have access and this location should be locked when unattended.[9]
- Outside working hours, fax machines should either be switched off or if left on should be locked away.
- Only use the fax machine when absolutely necessary as

  - the fax messages are not encrypted (unless such a module has been added and the same unit is used by the recipient machine)
  - the information could be intercepted or diverted
  - the transmission printout only confirms that the message left the fax machine but not its delivery (unless machines are directly connected)
  - there is no standard authentication method to verify the origin of the messages
  - output may be of low quality, risking misunderstanding
  - misdialling may send the fax message to a wrong machine.

- The risk of misdialling must be minimised. Measures to prevent this could be programming frequently used numbers into the fax machine, checking on a regular basis whether used numbers are up to date; always double-check whether numbers entered are correct before sending.
- Always confirm whether the fax has been received.
- When sending a fax ensure that only the minimum necessary patient-identifiable data is sent, and that the content of the fax is limited to the need-to-know basis.[2,8]
- Wherever possible clinical information should be sent without information with which a third party could easily identify the patient (name, address, DoB) but with a linking identifier (e.g. NHS number, hospital number or other local identifier).[13,14]
- The following faxing policy on the transfer of patient-identifiable information may be printed on your practice's letter-headed paper and distributed to all members of staff. You may wish to alter this policy to your specific needs.

- Ensure that your faxing policy meets the necessary local requirement. This insurance can be obtained from the Caldicott Guardian from your PCO.

Faxing policy
Guidance on the transfer of patient-identifiable information

(You might like to print the Faxing Policy from www.radcliffe-oxford.com/informationgov.)

The policy on the use of fax machines provides guidance on the handling and sending of facsimiles containing patient-identifiable information. This policy has been developed with reference to the Data Protection Act 1998, the common law duty of confidentiality, the Caldicott Principles[3] and EL(92)60.[12]

- The following outlines the steps to be taken when sending a fax:

    1 Ensure that the fax machine is operated in accordance with the manufacturer's instructions.
    2 Confirm if it is urgent and absolutely necessary to send the information by fax.
    3 Only fax a patient's identifiable information (name, address, date of birth) if any other means of identification (e.g. NHS number, hospital number) which a third/unauthorised party cannot easily identify cannot be used.
    4 Ensure that the fax contains the minimum necessary information to achieve its purpose.
    5 Ensure that highly sensitive information (e.g. HIV status) is not sent via fax.
    6 Confirm to whom the fax should be sent.
    7 Check if fax number is correct.
    8 Check if fax number has been entered correctly.
    9 Send a *cover sheet* (an example is provided after this policy) first, which

       – is clearly marked 'Confidential', as are all pages faxed
       – has contact details for the sender (or use your letter-headed paper)
       – shows clearly for whom the message is intended
       – contains the following message:

         The information in the fax is confidential. If you are *not* the above-named recipient of the fax, you are not authorised to read, keep, copy, alter or disclose the information of this fax as it is prohibited and may be unlawful. Please inform the sender (Tel _____) about this error and return the fax to the above address immediately.

    10 Check if the fax was received by the 'right' person.
    11 If a fax number will be used frequently, save it in the memory.
    12 Monitor transmission and obtain a printed record of transmission.
    13 All confidential faxes sent should be logged for future reference.

- A designated person, e.g. senior receptionist or secretary, should periodically check the validity of memory-stored or frequently used fax numbers.

- Any confidential facsimile received via the fax machines should be handled like any other confidential information received by the practice and the appropriate practice policies should be applied (e.g. policy on disclosure, records management, data ownership, security, access and so on).
- Every member of staff is obliged to report any potential or actual incident (*see* Section 15, Security incidents) if it occurs which should be logged and brought to the attention of the practice's Caldicott Guardian. Incidents include, for example:

  - mechanical failure
  - misdialling, disclosure to unauthorised person
  - poor quality printout
  - received faxes not handled according to the practice's policies.

- Any breach of this policy could lead to disciplinary action.

Cover sheet
Confidential and urgent

From Name: _____

Department/Address: _____

_____

_____

Tel: _____   Fax: _____

Date: ___ / ___ / ___   Time: _____

THIS FAX IS ONLY FOR THE ATTENTION OF:

To   Name: _____

Address: _____

_____

_____

Number of pages faxed: _____

The information in the fax is confidential. If you are *not* the above-named recipient of the fax, you are not authorised to read, keep, copy, alter or disclose the information of this fax as it is prohibited and may be unlawful. Please inform the sender about this error and return the fax to the above address immediately.

Disclosure Policy

Guidance on the disclosure of patient-identifiable information[1]

The disclosure policy gives guidance to every member of staff of a PHCT on disclosing patient data. (You might like to print this disclosure policy from www. radcliffe-oxford.com/informationgov.) It is essential for every member of the PHCT to understand that any disclosure of patient-identifiable information must be justified or otherwise constitutes a serious misconduct. Therefore the most important rule is

---

If you are in any doubt you must check with your line manager prior to disclosure of any patient-identifiable information!

When adopting a disclosure policy for your PHCT please ensure it meets your local requirements by seeking approval from the Caldicott Guardian of your PCO. The following questions should help in the decision-making process to determine if the disclosure of patient-identifiable information is justified.

Please answer these questions and follow the guidance to the answers before disclosing any patient-identifiable information.

Question 1

Are there any legal obligations or statutory requirements or any other reasons for which the consent to disclose patient-identifiable information is not needed, for example:

a   Is the disclosure necessary to fulfil a statutory obligation?
b   Is the disclosure necessary for the prevention, detection or prosecution of serious crime?
c   Is the disclosure necessary to fulfil a court order?
d   Is the disclosure necessary due to a significant public interest: i.e. prevention of a serious crime[15] or
e   protection of the public from a risk of serious disease (not including HIV)?
f   Is the disclosure necessary in the interest of the protection of children from abuse or harm?[16]
g   Has the disclosure been approved under Section 60 of the Health and Social Care Act 2001?

Answer:
> If any of the questions is answered YES, you must only disclose the information on a need-to-know basis. If you are unsure, ask your Caldicott Guardian. In some circumstances it might be necessary to seek legal advice. The patient should be informed about the disclosure and the reason for it, unless this would prejudge the outcome (e.g. prevention of a serious crime). In any case, the decision-making process and the advice sought must be well documented.

> If all the above questions are answered NO, please go to question 2.

Question 2
Have you got the consent for the disclosure of the patient's/client's confidential information?

a   Is the patient able to give consent or has his/her legal guardian given consent?
b   Was the complete (i.e. every item of confidential information) consent given explicitly and understood in its consequences?

Answer:
   If all the above questions are answered YES, please go to question 3.

   If NO to question 2a: If the patient/client is not able to give consent due to a life-threatening emergency then the Data Protection Act allows the sharing of patient-identifiable information. In any other case consent needs to be gained before disclosure.

   If NO to question 2b: The patient/client however might refuse consent or is only willing to give partial consent in which case the consequences of such refusal/partial refusal need to be understood by the patient/client. The patient/client may revoke his/her once-given consent or refusal of consent at any time. In any case the patient's/client's wishes have to be followed. Document this well!

Question 3
Does the disclosure involve any passing on of information about a third party?

Answer:
   If answered NO, please continue with question 4.

   If answered YES, this guidance should also be followed in respect to the third party or you might choose to erase any such references. This needs to be documented. If consent cannot be obtained but is deemed to be necessary, then as much information as possible without identifying the third party can be disclosed.

Question 4
Have the Caldicott Principles been adhered to for the proposed disclosure of information, e.g. is it on a strict need-to-know basis and does it give as little patient-identifiable information as possible?

Answer:
   If answered YES, please continue with question 5.

   If answered NO, please make sure before disclosure of the information that the Caldicott Principles have been applied and then go to question 5.

Question 5
Does the recipient of the information understand his/her duty to confidentiality and observe the same standard in the safeguarding of information as expected by NHS staff?

Answer:
   If answered YES – unless there are other relevant issues – send information to the recipient's safe haven.

If answered NO, the patient will need to be informed and further consent for this disclosure needs to be gained. You may also wish to discuss such matters with your Caldicott Guardian.

References

1   DoH (2003) *Confidentiality: NHS Code of Practice*, version 3.0. http://www. doh.gov.uk/ipu/confiden

2   DoH (1997) *The Caldicott Committee Report on the Review of Patient-identifiable Information*, December. http://www.hmso.gov.uk/confiden/app2.htm

3   DoH (1999) *Protecting and Using Patient Information: a manual for Caldicott Guardians. Protocols governing the receipt and disclosure of patient/client information*, March.

4   First Principle of the Data Protection Act 1998.

5   First Principle of the Data Protection Act 1998 and Article 8.1 of the Human Rights Act 1998: 'everyone has the right to respect for his private and family life, his home and his correspondence'.

6   First and Second Principle of the Data Protection Act 1998.

7   First and Seventh Principle of the Data Protection Act 1998. Exceptions where consent might not be required are detailed in schedule 2 and 3 of the Data Protection Act. Disclosure without consent might also be permitted, when the public good outweighs issues of privacy. Section 60 of the Health and Social Care Act 2001 provides further details when patient-identifiable information can be used without the consent of the patient.

8   Third Principle of the Data Protection Act 1998.

9   Seventh Principle of the Data Protection Act 1998.

10   First, Second and Seventh Principle of the Data Protection Act 1998.

11   *See* also NHSnet Code of Connection; NHS Information Authority Code of Connection; NHS Information Authority Security and Access Policy.

12   EL(92)60 issued in 1992: *Handling Confidential Patient Information in Contracting: a code of practice*.

13   EL(92)60: *Handling Confidential Patient Information in Contracting: a code of practice* suggests that if all the information needs to be sent (i.e. with either the patient's name or address or DoB) then confirmation should be sought after faxing the first part to ensure that the right person has received it before faxing the remainder. This appears to be currently not practical in the NHS.

14   The Caldicott Report recommendations 8 and 13 urge that wherever possible the new NHS number should replace other patient-identifiable information.

15   There is no clear definition of 'serious crime'. The General Medical Council (GMC) defined it as a crime that puts someone at risk of death or serious harm and would usually be a crime against the person, such as abuse of children (GMC guidance, *Confidentiality: protecting and providing information*). The definition of serious crime however may also need to take into consideration serious fraud or theft involving NHS resources. DoH (2003) *Confidentiality: NHS Code of Practice*. Section 115 of the Police and Criminal Evidence Act 1984 identifies 'Serious Arrestable Offences' as: treason, murder, manslaughter, rape, kidnapping, certain sexual offences, offences under the prevention of terrorism legislation, making a threat which if carried out would lead to a serious threat of security of the state or public order, serious interference with the administration of justice or with the investigation of an offence, death, serious financial loss to any person.

16   In considering the risk of harm not only the victim(s)' psychological and physical damage should be taken into account but also the effect it has on the victim(s)' relatives. DoH (2003) *Confidentiality: NHS Code of Practice*.

Section 3
Staff induction procedures

As outlined in the Preface of this *Toolkit*, confidentiality is a cornerstone in medical practice, i.e. in the relationship between doctor/PHCT and patient. Only when the patient is assured that his/her information is treated confidentially will the patient be able to seek help without fear that his/her rights of privacy, dignity and integrity are at risk.

The PHCTs have a legal responsibility to ensure that all patient information is handled properly.[1] The transfer of patient information and its collection must be performed with great care to ensure patient confidentiality. The Data Protection Act 1998 (*see* Chapter 2) places the responsibility on the data controllers (i.e. your PCHT) to handle patient information appropriately, i.e. within the provisions of the law.[2]

All new members of staff should be made aware of their duties and responsibilities at the commencement of their employment.

Therefore it is very important that every member of staff is familiar and complies with the law and the policies that aim to ensure patient confidentiality and information security, which are covered by the following core topics in this book:

- Staff code of conduct[3] (*see* Chapter 4, p. 131)
- Principles of Data Protection Act 1998 (*see* Chapter 2)
- Caldicott Principles[4]
- IM&T training (*see* Chapter 4, p. 132)
- security policy (*see* Chapter 4, p. 140)[5,6]
- user responsibilities (*see* Chapter 4, p. 142)[7]
- safe-haven procedures (*see* Chapter 4, p. 138).[8]

It might be prudent to document that every member of staff has been made aware and given a copy of all the above-mentioned laws and policies. It is also important at this stage to determine the level of access to confidential information and fill in the form: 'Registration of IM&T system users' (*see* Section 18, Access controls).

Compliance with the named policies should be part of staff appraisals and of the assessment for training needs (*see* Section 4).

The following form gives a checklist of topics to be covered in staff induction procedures and a signed copy should be kept in the personal file of the employee.

You might like to print this checklist from www.radcliffe-oxford.com/informationgov.

Staff induction procedures
Checklist

Name: _____

Job title: _____

Date: ____/____/____

Topics: (please tick box when training is completed)

Staff code of conduct ☐

Principles of Data Protection Act 1998 ☐

Caldicott Principles ☐

IM&T training ☐

Security policy ☐

User responsibilities ☐

Safe-haven procedures ☐

Access level to confidential data determined ☐

Training provision agreed _____

_____

I have had explained and received a copy of the above principles, policies and procedures.

Signature of employee: _____

Signature of practice's Caldicott Guardian: _____
(Practice manager/GP)

References

1   The First Principle of the Data Protection Act (DPA) puts the obligations on NHS/PHCT staff to ensure that patient-identifiable information is processed fairly and lawfully. The word 'processing' in the DPA is defined as holding, obtaining, using, recording, disclosure or destruction of information which applies to any form of media, i.e. paper, computer record or images on videos etc. Except for few exemptions any processing of patient-identifiable information requires the explicit consent of the patient, which is only gained if the patient understands the reason for its processing, who handles and has access to his/her information and to whom it might be disclosed. For further information *see* Chapter 2 in this book or *see* http://www.dataprotection.gov.uk. Besides the DPA there is the common law of confidentiality which over a long period of time has been established by case law. The Human Rights Act 1998 in Article 8 – right to 'respect for private and family life' – puts an emphasis on the right to privacy of individuals.

2   Seventh Principle of the Data Protection Act 1998.

3   DoH (2003) *Confidentiality: NHS Code of Practice*, version 3.0. http://www.doh. gov.uk/ipu/confiden

4   DoH (1999) *Protecting and Using Patient Information: a manual for Caldicott Guardians. Protocols governing the receipt and disclosure of patient/client information*, March.

5   NHS Executive's Security and Data Protection Programme (1999) *Ensuring Security and Confidentiality in NHS Organisations: protecting the security of information in NHS organisations*, IMG Ref No E5501.

6   BS 7799-1:1999: *Information Security Management – Part 1: Code of practice for information security management*. http://www.nhsia.nhs.uk/erdip/pages/docs_ egif/evaluation/technical/ehr-req-final.pdf

7   NHS Executive's Security and Data Protection Programme (1999) *Play IT Safe: a practical guide to IT security for everyone working in general practice*, version 1.1. Available from the NHS Information Authority.

8   EL(92)60 issued in 1992: *Handling Confidential Patient Information in Contracting: a code of practice*.

Section 4
Confidentiality and security training needs

The GP or Caldicott Guardian/Information Governance Lead of the PCHT is obliged to assess and make sure that the appropriate and necessary training for practice staff is delivered.[1]

Training needs should be assessed regularly, and a yearly training in and updating on confidentiality and security issues is recommended.

Special awareness and training for every member of staff is needed on issues of disclosure of confidential information, especially that consent is obtained if patient-identifiable information is used for purposes other than direct patient care or when disclosure is permitted despite the patient not giving explicit consent (e.g. section 60 of the Health and Social Care Act 2001, schedule 2 and 3 of the Data Protection Act 1998, Crime and Disorder Act 1998, Children's Act 1989).[2]

Training needs of staff members will differ depending on their role and responsibilities in respect of processing and collecting confidential personal information. The Caldicott Guardian/Information Governance Lead will need special ongoing training to keep up to date.

The following checklist, therefore, is just a guide to topics that could be relevant. You might like to print this checklist on training needs from www.radcliffe-oxford.com/informationgov.

Assessment of confidentiality and security training needs

Checklist

Name: _____

Job title: _____

	Date of last training	Training needed
		Yes No
Access controls (Section 18)	/ /	☐ ☐
Caldicott Principles	/ /	☐ ☐
IT skills up to date	/ /	☐ ☐
Other law/legal requirements	/ /	☐ ☐
Other practice protocols	/ /	☐ ☐
Principles of Data Protection Act 1998	/ /	☐ ☐
Safe-haven procedures (Section 10)	/ /	☐ ☐
Security policy (Section 12)	/ /	☐ ☐
Security responsibilities (Section 13)	/ /	☐ ☐
Staff code of conduct (Section 2)	/ /	☐ ☐
User responsibilities (Section 17)	/ /	☐ ☐
Data quality/PRIMIS	/ /	☐ ☐

Further issues:

_____

Action plan: _____

_____

Signature of employee: _____ Date: __/__/__

Signature of assessor: _____ Date: __/__/__
(Practice's Caldicott Guardian/practice manager/GP)

References

1   Seventh Principle of the Data Protection Act 1998.
2   First Principle of the Data Protection Act 1998.

Section 5
Communication with patients/information for patients

The First Principle of the Data Protection Act 1998 requires that 'personal data shall be processed fairly' by the data controller.[1] Although the word 'fairly' is not further defined in the Act it is certain that unless the patient receives all necessary information about the uses of his or her data the processing of such data can not be fair.[2] Besides the Data Protection Act, the Caldicott requirements[3] as well as guidance from the DoH[4] also demand that patients are informed about the use of their confidential information. This section of the book first outlines the basic principles on what type of information the patient should be supplied with, secondly gives suggestions on a communication strategy and the dialogue with the patient to achieve these requirements, and thirdly suggests questions for a patient survey to assess the effectiveness in achieving these requirements.

Basic principles[2]

1   According to the Data Protection Act every patient should receive 'fair processing information' when his/her personal data are processed. This means that the data subject (i.e. an individual such as a patient, client, carer, relative) must understand: who is the data controller, the proposed use(s) of his or her personal data, who else will get to know (i.e. to whom the personal data will be disclosed) and any other necessary information which is specifically relevant to the processing of his or her personal data.

2   The patient/data subject needs to be able to exercise his/her rights in relation to how his/her data are, or are to be, processed and be able to assess the risks to him or her in providing that data or not.[5]

3   The information provided by the PHCT should enable the patient to make an informed decision (*see* also Chapter 2, Individuals' rights). To achieve that, the PHCT should strike a balance between being too general or too detailed or giving an unnecessary amount of information or too little information. It is important for the patient to understand the implications of sharing or not sharing his/her personal data. The information the PHCT provides must be objective and honest.

4   Furthermore, to give an informed consent the patient must know which data about him/her exist, when information is recorded and who will have access to the record. Only then can the patient's consent be informed as to the way these data may be processed. It is therefore important that the patient is given every opportunity to read through his/her record and that the patient has got no concerns or queries about how his or her information is used.

5   The patient should be involved and be allowed to make choices. He/she should be aware that choices are available in respect of the use or sharing of his/her information. A process must be in place ensuring that patients' wishes are responded to and that patients' wishes are accurately taken into account. Especially the practice has to ensure that an informed consent has been given before personal details are processed (unless special circumstances apply).

6   The patient must be told that his/her consent can be withdrawn in the future (including any difficulties in withdrawing information that has already been disclosed).

7   The patient might need to know who the typical NHS bodies are with whom information might be shared, or to whom transferred/disclosed, or by whom used/handled (i.e. typical data flows). He/she should know when his/her information may or will be shared with others.

8   The patient should be reminded from time to time how the information is being used.

9   Certain information which is specific for special circumstances should be given in context and at the relevant time (e.g. patient information passed on to the cancer register, or information passed on due to adverse drug reaction).

10   The way information is communicated has to take into account special circumstances, for example the level of understanding, command of the English language and sensitivity of the data.

11   Systems should be in place which ensure a high level of data quality. Patient data should only be processed if they are accurate, up to date, relevant and not excessive in relation to the purpose(s)[6] (*see* data quality of records in Section 10, Safe-haven procedures).

12   Although the use of patient-identifiable information without consent is allowed in certain circumstances (e.g. section 60 of the Health and Social Care Act 2001)[7] the First Principle of the Data Protection Act 1998 still requires that fair processing information should be given to the patient. The only exemptions to this rule are situations where providing 'fair processing information' might prejudice the purpose (e.g. for the detection of fraud, malpractice and so on – i.e. if section 29 or 31 of the Data Protection Act applies).

Communication strategy

The PHCT is obliged to provide fair processing information.[8] This process may be integrated with existing procedures, unless circumstances arise that require specific communication.

The ways of communication could be through

1   patient information leaflets
2   posters
3   other means such as face-to-face conversation or letter.

The practice should have procedures in place to answer difficult patient questions regarding the processing of his/her information. It would be advisable that a senior member of staff (for example the Caldicott Guardian) is responsible for such requests, acknowledges the receipt as well as responds to it in a given timeframe and using the preferred means (verbal, letter, email) of communication agreed on with the applicant.

Patient information leaflets[9]

To fulfil this legal requirement an example of an information leaflet has been designed in this section, 'Protecting and using your personal and medical information'.

This or a similar leaflet should be readily available in the practice for patients/clients. It would be ideal to make this (or a shorter version of it) a part of the practice leaflet.

The leaflet gives guidance as to what the patient/client should be informed about. It only provides the core information; however, it can be amended and extended. The practice should have procedures in place to review on an annual basis if the information provided in the leaflet is accurate and up to date covering the purposes for which patient data are used. A final section in the leaflet could inform the patients/clients about the access to confidential information and the responsibilities of each member of staff in your PHCT regarding confidential information, e.g.:

- Receptionist has access to medical records to organise repeat prescriptions, 'Read code' information from discharge/hospital letters, tag case notes, file hospital letters or correspondence and laboratory results, take details for home visits.
- Secretary has access to medical records to type referral letters, for the filing of letters/correspondence, to 'Read code'.
- Practice manager has access similar to that of a receptionist and secretary.

Finally, once a suitable wording of the leaflet for the PHCT has been found, this leaflet should then be translated according to the needs of minorities and made suitable for reading by disabled clients/patients.[8]

A draft version of a poster about confidentiality aims to make patients/clients aware that some confidential information has to be passed on.

As some patient-related data is passed to the PCO, the PCO will develop its own 'patient information leaflet', which may be handed out together with the practice leaflet. Both leaflets will complement each other and improve the knowledge of the patient and the transparency of how his or her personal data are handled within the NHS.

The box suggests a wording that could be used as part of a practice leaflet and you can print this leaflet from www.radcliffe-oxford.com/informationgov.

Protecting and using your personal and medical information

Introduction
All the information you give to a member of the PHCT (e.g. doctor, practice or district nurse, health visitor) which is held either on paper records or computer is safeguarded by the Data Protection Act 1998. This Act sets clear rules about how the recorded information can be used and demands openness about how the information is used. It also gives you certain rights, e.g. you have the right of access to your health records. If you want to see your record you should write to us. You have the right to receive a copy of your record but usually you will have to pay for this.

At all times, everybody working for the NHS – i.e. all the members of the PHCT – has a legal duty to keep information about you confidential.

Why do we need information about you?
We have to ask you for information so that we can make a decision about the best care and treatment for your needs.

This information and the information about the care you receive are often kept on paper record or on computer because we might need it when we see you again or you have questions about your care or treatment.

Your record will include your:

- name, address, date of birth, telephone number and next of kin
- allergies
- treatments, for example your tablets and medicines
- jabs/immunisations against diseases or illnesses like tetanus, flu, whooping cough, polio
- information from other health professionals such as nurses, health visitors, physiotherapists
- results of tests such as x-rays and blood tests.

What else do we do with this information?
In some cases the GP has to pass on information about your treatment or care so the practice can get paid for it. GPs declare when cervical screening and certain childhood vaccinations have been performed. Your GP might need to ask the PCT to fund certain elements of your care and for this we may need to give the PCT details of your personal and clinical records.

The GP needs to notify the PCT when you first register and your entire health record will be sent to the PCT when you change your GP. The PCT will then pass these records over to your new GP.

If you are referred to a specialist (e.g. consultant) or need assistance in your treatment or management (e.g. require a wheelchair, need help from social services, counselling etc.) relevant information about you will be passed on so we can all work together for your benefit.

The information is also used for doctors and nurses/health professionals who are learning about health and treatments.

Sometimes other people are allowed to look at your health records without asking you
- The law demands that details of patients with certain serious infectious diseases that can spread, like measles or meningitis, have to be passed on to the authorities so action can be taken to protect the public's health. You can receive a list of all notifiable diseases from the PCT.
- The law demands that information is passed on if a serious crime (e.g. murder, manslaughter, rape, child abuse, kidnapping) can be prevented.
- When a baby is born the registrar working for the government must be told.
- If you are not well and are a danger to yourself or others, doctors and nurses might have to tell other people who can help you to keep you safe and get the right treatments for you.
- Information about you may also be needed to review the care you receive to make sure it is of the highest standard. It is used for the managing and planning of the NHS, so that services can meet patient needs in the future, accounts can be audited and the NHS performance and activity analysed.

However, we will only pass information on to people who really need to know it and have a genuine interest and we also will only pass on as much information as is absolutely necessary.

> You can choose whether or not to be involved in the training and education of staff or students and if you want to participate in clinical trials or other research projects.
>
> *Anyone to whom information about you is passed by a member of this practice is also under a legal duty to keep it confidential.*
>
> Partner organisations with whom information about you may be shared are:
>
> - strategic health authority [name]
> - PCT [name]
> - NHS trusts [names of hospitals]
> - ambulance service [name]
> - social services
> - education services
> - voluntary and private sector providers [names].
>
> *Without your authorisation we cannot pass on information about the progress of your health to your relatives, friends and carers.*
>
> If you would like further information please do not hesitate to contact:
>
> [name] [job title] [address] [tel] [email].

Posters

Displaying posters in the surgery is a means of raising awareness of patients, carers and relatives on how the practice handles patient information and patients' rights of access to their information. A poster is not deemed to be enough as the only route of communication.[2] It should be seen as only a part of an information strategy which is supported by other initiatives of communication such as leaflets and explanations provided during a consultation. The following suggests the wording of a poster which you might like to print from www.radcliffe-oxford.com/informationgov and display in your surgery.

> Everyone working in this practice and for the NHS has a legal duty to keep information about you confidential.
>
> Sometimes we have to pass your information on, but anyone who receives this information is also under a legal duty to keep this information confidential.
>
> If you want to know more about your rights and our legal duties in handling confidential information, please ask for a leaflet about confidentiality at the reception desk.

Other means such as face-to-face conversation or letter

Uses of patient information not covered in the patient information leaflet should be discussed with the data subject (i.e. the patient, relative or carer to whom the data is related) either during the consultation or by letter. Consultations should also be used to remind patients of the use(s) of their data and to check the data subject's understanding of the processing of personal data. Sometimes information on the processing of data only becomes relevant to a patient in special circumstances, for example the diagnosis of cancer and the disclosure of patient data to the cancer register.

The PHCT should nominate a person who can handle difficult questions about the processing of data.

Patient surveys

It is important for the PHCT to assess if its information strategy achieves its purpose. A possible way of determining this is by using patient surveys. With patient surveys you can not only elicit the effectiveness but also the patients' satisfaction with the information strategy. Useful questions might be:

- Does the patient know who processes and what type of personal data are processed as well as how these are processed by the PHCT?
- Is sufficient information provided by the PHCT for the patient in order for him/ her to give an informed consent?
- Is your method of distributing this information to the patients sufficient?
- Does the practice leaflet need changing?
- Have patients' choices been taken into account to the patients' satisfaction?

Results of a patient survey may influence your information governance strategy (*see* Section 20) and, for example, change the way you communicate with your patients by changing the content of the leaflet or poster or the way in which you distribute them.

References

1   The First Principle of the Data Protection Act puts the obligation on NHS/ PHCT staff to ensure that patient-identifiable information is processed fairly and lawfully. For further information *see* Chapter 2 in this book or *see* http:// www.dataprotection.gov.uk.

2   Information Commissioner (2002) *Use and Disclosure of Health Data: guidance on the application of the Data Protection Act 1998*, May. http://www.information commissioner.gov.uk

3   DoH (1999) *Protecting and Using Patient Information: a manual for Caldicott Guardians. Protocols governing the receipt and disclosure of patient/client information*, March. http://www.hmso.gov.uk/confiden/app2.htm, Annex A.

4   DoH (2003) *Confidentiality: NHS Code of Practice*, version 3.0. http://www. doh.gov.uk/ipu/confiden

5   'Processed' is defined as any activity undertaken with the information or data such as obtaining, recording or holding, or carrying out any operation or set of operations. *See* also Chapter 2.

6 Third and Fourth Principle of the Data Protection Act 1998.
7 Only applicable in England and Wales.
8 First Principle of the Data Protection Act 1998.
9 DoH (1999) *Protecting and Using Patient Information: a manual for Caldicott Guardians.*

Section 6
Staff contracts

All members of the PHCT who will have access to confidential information should sign a confidentiality undertaking.[1-3] This includes attached staff and anybody who works within or for the surgery, even if only on a temporary basis, and may therefore have the potential to get in contact with confidential information.[4]

Prior to signing the confidentiality undertaking the signing party should understand his/her obligations and responsibilities in safeguarding confidentiality.[5] It might be prudent to let the staff member sign a clause specifically mentioning that the Principles of the Data Protection Act and Caldicott and security policy (*see* Section 12) have been carefully explained and understood. It will be useful to use the checklist for staff induction procedures (*see* Section 3).

Confidentiality undertakings should be reviewed on a regular basis especially if the terms of contract of a staff member and/or the job description change since this might affect the level of access to sensitive data.

Particular attention should be given to situations when contracts are terminated so that e.g. keys are returned, passwords invalidated and computer access is denied in the future (*see* Section 18, Access controls).

The following text suggests a wording to be used in staff contracts. You might like to print this wording from www.radcliffe-oxford.com/informationgov.

I understand that during the course of my employment/attachment, I may have access to confidential information about patients, their carers, members of staff or other health service business. This should be handled as strictly confidential at all times — even after the termination of employment/attachment. On no account should patient-identifiable and confidential information be disclosed to anyone other than those persons whom the patient consented to have their information passed on to (i.e. authorised persons, for example medical, nursing or other staff as appropriate who are involved with the care, diagnosis and/or treatment of the patient) unless specific conditions apply which would authorise the disclosure in pursuit of my duties or through authorisation of my line manager.

I understand my duty of confidentiality and I will at all times adhere to the security policy and other policies of this practice (e.g. staff code of conduct, safe-haven procedures, health records management) and comply with my obligations and responsibilities in safeguarding confidentiality.

(A further paragraph might be added which details certain duties specific to the job role of a member of staff, e.g. the person in charge of computer backup tapes, not to share passwords, etc.)

I understand that failure to observe my duty to confidentiality will result in disciplinary action being taken against me, including possibly dismissal and legal proceedings.

Signature: _____   Date: /   /

References

1 DoH (1999) *Protecting and Using Patient Information: a manual for Caldicott Guardians. Management audits and improvement plans*, March.
2 DoH (2003) *Confidentiality: NHS Code of Practice*, version 3.0. http://www. doh.gov.uk/ipu/confiden
3 Seventh Principle of the Data Protection Act 1998.
4 For further guidance *see* also: ISO/IEC 17799:2000(E); BS 7799-1:2000.
5 First and Second Principle of the Data Protection Act 1998.

Section 7
Contracts placed with other organisations

Non-NHS agencies might be contracted to carry out specific tasks, e.g. cleaning, removal of clinical waste, maintenance of computer systems, building work and the like.

It is the responsibility of the practice to[1]

- ensure that everybody employed by the practice understands the need for confidentiality, and maintains it
- ensure that systems and mechanisms are in place to protect confidentiality
- ensure that contracts with non-NHS agencies/individuals specify appropriate confidentiality and security requirements of the same standard as is expected for best practice in NHS organisations, especially in terms of patient confidentiality.[2,3] The more contractors are exposed to sensitive/confidential information the tighter the controls on their activities should be and the stricter their specification of qualifications should be (e.g. registration under the Data Protection Act) to perform the work.

It is important that these non-NHS agencies either have a clause in the contracts or sign a separate confidentiality undertaking.

The following pages give an example of the wording of a confidentiality agreement for contractors[4] and an agreement for their employees. You might like to print the wording of this confidentiality agreement from www.radcliffe-oxford. com/informationgov on your practice's letter-headed paper. You may wish to alter this confidentiality agreement to your specific needs. In doing so, please ensure that the agreement meets the necessary requirements.

Confidentiality agreement with contractor

Confidentiality Agreement (contractor)

The contractor ensures that he/she, all his/her employees and those of the subcontractor

1 will treat *all* information which may be derived from or be obtained in the course of the work performed for the contract or as a result of it as strictly confidential and
2 will provide all the necessary safety measures to guarantee that all such information remains confidential
3 shall not disclose or use such information in any unlawful manner
4 will continue to observe the duty to confidentiality after fulfilment/termination of the contract
5 will adhere to the provisions of the Data Protection Act 1998 and the security standards outlined in BS 7799
6 will indemnify the practice against any loss arising under the Data Protection Act 1998 through action, taken by himself/herself, his/her employees or subcontractors, irrespective of whether the action was authorised or unauthorised.

In the event of a breach of confidentiality the contract may be terminated immediately.

Only in exceptional circumstances may information be disclosed under the Public Interest Disclosure Act 1998.

The organisation agrees to adhere to the insurances set out above. All employees and those of the subcontractor are obliged to sign a confidentiality agreement prior to access to the practice's premises.

The organisation is appropriately registered under the Data Protection Act 1998 and is legally entitled to undertake the specified work in the contract agreed with the practice (cross out if not applicable).

Company/Organisation: _____

Address: _____

_____

Postcode: _____   Tel: (_____) _____

Name
(PRINT): _____
(signing on behalf of the company/organisation)

Position: _____
(within the company/organisation)

Signature: _____   Date: / / _____

Authorised by (on behalf of the practice)

Name
(PRINT): _____

Position: _____
(Practice's Caldicott Guardian/practice manager/GP)

Signed: _____   Date: / / _____

Confidentiality agreement for employees of the contractor/subcontractor

You might like to print this agreement from www.radcliffe-oxford.com/informationgov on your letter-headed paper.

Confidentiality Agreement (employees of contractor or subcontractor)

I understand that *any* information about a person (e.g. name, address, date of birth, sex, religion, medical or social details) or business information of this practice that I might acquire during the pursuit of the work carried out for the contract is strictly confidential and that it is my duty not to disclose this information to anybody. In an event of a breach of confidentiality the contract may be terminated immediately.

I understand that any breaches of confidentiality associated with the terms of the Data Protection Act 1998 could result in legal action against me and my employer.

Name
(PRINT): _____

Position: _____

Company/Organisation: _____

Address: _____

_____

Postcode: _____ Tel: (_____) _____

Signed: _____ Date: _/_ /_

References

1 Seventh Principle of the Data Protection Act 1998.
2 DoH (1999) *Protecting and Using Patient Information: a manual for Caldicott Guardians. Protocols governing the receipt and disclosure of patient/client information*, March.
3 NHS Executive's Security and Data Protection Programme (1999) *Ensuring Security and Confidentiality in NHS Organisations: protecting the security of information in NHS organisations*, IMG Ref No E5501.
4 Based on a clause from *Introduction to Data Protection in the NHS* (E5127) and BS 7799. Please refer to *Introduction to Data Protection in the NHS* (E5127) for confidentiality agreements involving contractors dealing with, for example, computer hardware and software which contains person-identifiable information.

Section 8
Reviewing information flows

The Caldicott Report requests that every flow (i.e. sharing, transfer, disclosure, use, handling) of patient-identifiable information/data within and from the PHCT should be checked against the Caldicott Principles,[1] which are as follows:

Principle 1: Justify the purpose(s) for using confidential information.
Principle 2: Only use confidential information when absolutely necessary.
Principle 3: Use the minimum of information that is required.
Principle 4: Access to the information should be on a strict need-to-know basis.
Principle 5: Everyone must understand his/her responsibilities.
Principle 6: Understand the law and comply with it.

By improving the security and confidentiality of information flows (*see* Section 12) as well as by adapting the Caldicott Principles to the information flow the patient's privacy can be enhanced.[2] These measures will lessen the chances of a patient being inadvertently recognised. Provided that the Data Protection Act 1998 has been complied with, the improvement in privacy that would be gained by removing data items should outweigh the cost, risk and impact of making that change.

The aims of reviewing information flows are:

- to verify that each patient-identifying data is serving a necessary purpose in the information flow and
- to reduce the patient-identifiable data in a flow to the minimum necessary.[3]

Patient-identifiable information/data, which should be justified in their use, are:

- forename
- surname
- date of birth
- sex
- address
- postcode.

To assist in applying the general Caldicott Principles to the data flows a set of rules for reviewing patient-identifiable data flows has been established, published in *Protecting and Using Patient Information, a manual for Caldicott Guardians*:

Rule 1   Personal data should not be excessive for their purpose.
Rule 2   Wherever possible names and addresses should be retrieved locally — if there is a 'need-to-know'.
Rule 3   Where identifiable data are needed to trace a patient, the transfer of name and address may be justified in the short term.
Rule 4   Flows should be prioritised for change in which the confidentiality gain outweighs the risk and cost of the change.

Rule 5 In cases where the cost of changing a flow exceeds the benefits or is unreasonable, consider the removal of name and address once the data have reached the recipient.

Although every information flow (i.e. sharing, transfer, disclosure, use, handling) with patient-identifiable information should be reviewed, there are, however, two main areas, which should be carefully looked at:

1 *Patient care services*, which include healthcare teams providing mental health, community and acute services through doctors, nurses and paramedical professionals, social services and which applies to all service areas where care is provided directly to patients. Most transfer/sharing/disclosure of information will be justified; however, there may be some flows that do not relate directly to patient care and these flows should be reviewed, especially flows to:

• support research and audit
• public health
• voluntary bodies (e.g. patient support groups)
• and from other organisations
• information and contracting organisations.

2 *PCO/GP communications*, which include all data flows that support the delivery of primary care, such as:

• the managing and planning of services
• auditing of performance
• monitoring and protecting public health
• investigation of complaints
• risk management.

These areas of review should only take place together with the PCO and will become more relevant with the increase in computerisation of GP practices.

For each review, the person responsible for reviewing data flows should print off and answer the following questionnaire,[4] which will help to assist and structure the review procedure and helps the decision making if any information flow holds more patient data than needed and which patient-identifiable information should be omitted or changed.

There are many options that can be considered to change the flow (e.g. re-designing forms, improving the security of the flow, stopping or splitting the flow to make sure only the very necessary data reach the recipient).

However, before changing an information flow (i.e. sharing, transfer, disclosure, use, handling of information) a proposal should be drawn up taking into account the cost implication and practicability of such a change. Finally agreement should be sought with the sender, recipient(s), other PHCTs and the Caldicott Guardian of the PCO. The PCO's Caldicott Guardian might need to consider how to use these findings to improve the information-sharing protocols (*see* Section 11) with other organisations.

You might like to print this form from www.radcliffe-oxford.com/information gov.

Reviewing information flows

Review of information flow (i.e. sharing/transfer/disclosure/use/handling of information) performed by:

Name: _____

Job title: _____

Date completed: _____ / ___ / _____

Question 1
What was the purpose of the data flow?

_____

_____

_____

_____

_____

_____

Question 2
Who or which organisation initiates this data flow?

_____

_____

_____

_____

_____

_____

Question 3

What type(s) of patient-identifiable data items are used in this data flow you review? Please indicate:

☐ forename	☐ surname	☐ initials
☐ sex	☐ address	☐ postcode
☐ date of birth	☐ other dates/death	☐ ethnic group
☐ NHS number	☐ NI number	☐ local identifier
☐ other not listed above:		

Question 4

Please specify for which purpose(s) the patient-identifiable data items in the data flow you review were used.

A   Patient contact
B   Patient visit or correspondence
C   Confirmation of address/residency
D   Decision making about the patient's care
E   Creating or updating a patient record
F   Statutory requirements
G   Merger of existing patient data sets/correspondence

Any other purposes: _____

_____

The following table lists the recommended uses of patient-identifiable information for each purpose:

	Purpose for requiring patient-identifiable information	*Recommended uses of patient-identifiable information to achieve the purpose*
A	Patient contact	Name
B	Patient visit or correspondence	Name, address, NHS number, postcode
C	Confirmation of address/residency	Postcode
D	Decision making about the patient's care	DoB
E	Creating or updating a patient record	Name, address, postcode, DoB
F	Statutory requirements	Name, address, DoB, NHS number
G	Merger of existing patient data sets/correspondence	NHS number, DoB, postcode

Question 5

After you compared the patient-identifiable information you review in the data flow with the recommended uses in the table above, please state if the use of all patient-identifiable information in the data flow you review is justified.

Answer: _____

Question 6

Please state if the information flow you review allows the possibilities of minimising the use of patient-identifiable data or reducing the possibility of patient identification and still achieving its purpose, e.g.

a   by omission of some of the patient-identifiable information:

_____

b   by the use of local identifiers, which can only be obtained locally:

_____

_____

Question 7

If some of the patient-identifiable information could be omitted, please specify which items are possibly not justified.

☐ forename	☐ surname	☐ initials
☐ sex	☐ address	☐ postcode
☐ date of birth	☐ other dates/death	☐ ethnic group
☐ NHS number	☐ NI number	☐ local identifier
☐ other not listed above:		

Question 8

What might be the implications if this data flow would remove certain patient-identifiable information you have identified as unjustified?

a   risk of not properly identifying a patient:

_____

_____

_____

_____

_____

b   estimated cost implication:

_____

_____

_____

Question 9
Having discussed the possible implications of removing unjustified patient-identifiable information from the data flow with your PHCT and PCO's Caldicott Guardian/Information Governance Lead, what is the outcome?

_____

_____

_____

_____

_____

_____

_____

Signature: _____
(Practice's Caldicott Guardian/practice manager/GP)

Please file this review for future reference.

References

1   DoH (1997) *The Caldicott Committee Report on the Review of Patient-identifiable Information*, December. http://www.hmso.gov.uk/confiden/app2.htm. Also the Third Principle of the Data Protection Act 1998 requires that personal data held for any purpose(s) should be adequate, relevant and not excessive in relation to that/those purpose(s).
2   Seventh Principle of the Data Protection Act 1998.
3   Third Principle of the Data Protection Act 1998.
4   The questionnaire is an adaptation from the questionnaire published in: DoH (1999) *Protecting and Using Patient Information: a manual for Caldicott Guardians. Reviewing information flows*, March.

Section 9
Information/data 'ownership'

The wording of data 'ownership' might be misleading as it could be argued that the real owner of information is the patient him-/herself. However, all the information that is gathered from patients and is kept either in manual or on computer records needs to have an 'owner' within the PHCT who takes ultimate responsibility for all these confidential data.

In a single-handed practice the GP should have the overall data 'ownership' of all the confidential data. But in a partnership or group practice one GP/Caldicott Guardian should be assigned to have the overall responsibility for all the confidential data.[1,2]

For security purposes, however, each set of confidential data and/or material should be assigned/delegated to an 'owner'. For example, the GP/Caldicott Guardian is the overall data owner who delegates the data ownership of case notes and computer/electronically held data in the reception area to the senior receptionist; the senior secretary is given the data ownership of confidential data in the office; the practice nurse is entrusted with the data ownership of all confidential data present in her treatment room and so on. Counsellors, district nurses and health visitors who hold their own confidential records have the data ownership of these data.

The main responsibility of the data 'owner' is to keep these data as confidential as possible by[3]

- *working closely with the practice's Caldicott Guardian/Information Governance Lead*
- *identifying confidential data* (e.g. records, computers, backup tapes, letters/mail, fax machines) *and determining their sensitivity level to grant access to them accordingly*[4]
- *ensuring that only those data are kept that serve a justified purpose*[5]
- *specifying how the data should be used*[4] (this also includes that the copying, archiving or dumping of any data should be authorised by the data owner)
- *agreeing who is allowed to have access to these confidential data*[6,7] (*see* also Section 18, Access controls)
- *making sure that these data are as well secured as possible*[7] (*see* also Section 12, Security policy)
- *ensuring compliance with relevant legislation.*[4]

The following gives an example of a register of data 'owners'.

Register of data 'ownership'

Confidential data:	Data 'owner'	Signature
Reception area	_____	_____
Consultation room 1	_____	_____
Consultation room 2	_____	_____
Treatment room	_____	_____
Secretary's room	_____	_____
Practice manager's room	_____	_____
Storing cabinets	_____	_____
Backup tapes	_____	_____
Computer software and hardware	_____	_____

The data 'owner' – by signing this form – agrees to take over the responsibility for the data sets he/she 'owns', and to work closely with the practice's Caldicott Guardian.

Review date: ____/____/____

Authorised by (signature): _____
(Practice's Caldicott Guardian/practice manager/GP)

Date: ____/____/____

References

1 HSC 1999/012: *Caldicott Guardians*.
2 DoH (1999) *Protecting and Using Patient Information: a manual for Caldicott Guardians*, March.
3 NHS Executive's Security and Data Protection Programme (1999) *Ensuring Security and Confidentiality in NHS Organisations: protecting the security of information in NHS organisations*, IMG Ref No E5501.
4 First and Second Principle of the Data Protection Act 1998.
5 Second and Third Principle of the Data Protection Act 1998.
6 Seventh Principle of the Data Protection Act 1998.
7 First and Seventh Principle of the Data Protection Act 1998.

Section 10
Safe-haven procedures

Part of the information governance requirement is to have safe-haven procedures in place.[1,2] The term 'safe-haven procedures' stands for a set of administrative arrangements designed to ensure the safety and secure handling of confidential patient information.[3] This includes having one designated contact point per physical site through which all confidential information is to be disclosed or accepted.

These procedures must cover:

1 management arrangements
2 the staff responsible for managing the information
3 the physical location of offices/room and devices for the receiving, storing and handling of information
4 staff access to information in their work
5 the procedures for the handling of information
6 the receiving of information
7 the disclosure of information
8 the storage of information
9 the archiving and destroying of information
10 the use of computer systems.

Points 4, 5, 7, 8 and 9 form part of a records management policy. It is an information governance requirement for a general practice to have a policy on records management.

The following paragraphs intend to explain each of the above points and at the end of this section there will be an example of a records management policy.

1 *Management arrangements*
   Someone in the practice should be responsible for ensuring that confidentiality is maintained, procedures safeguarding confidentiality are adhered to, and that security of confidential information is guaranteed. The most likely person would be the person designated to have 'data ownership' (*see* Section 9) or the practice's Caldicott Guardian. All members of staff should be aware of the existence of safe-haven policies and procedures. All policies and procedures should be reviewed regularly (yearly) with regard to their effectiveness.

2 *The staff responsible for managing the information*
   Whatever level of access the member of staff has, it is important that any handling of confidential information only takes place on a strict need-to-know basis and only as part of his/her legitimate activity to fulfil his/her job requirements[3] (for further information *see* Section 2, Staff code of conduct).
   All members of staff who are allowed access to confidential information have to understand the law and comply with it (*see* Chapter 2, Data Protection Act).

3 *The physical location of offices and devices for the receiving, storing and handling of information*
   The physical location of a 'safe haven' must be clearly identifiable, physically secure, i.e. a lockable room, and access should preferably be via one entry

point so that access can be easily controlled. In most practices the 'safe haven' would be the room where all patient records are stored. However, where not every unit that holds confidential information can be located in one secure area (e.g. computers in different consultation rooms), then these 'stand-alone' units and the rooms where they are located would need to be treated as safe-haven areas and be subject to the same safe-haven procedures.

Confidential information should only be disclosed or accepted through designated safe-haven contact points (e.g. an area in the reception where all the mail, faxes, green bag and message book are kept). Confidential information should only be disclosed through a designated safe-haven point to a similar point in another organisation.

This secured physical location or 'safe-haven' should be used to hold the maximum possible confidential information, i.e. incoming/outgoing post, fax machines, computer systems, backup tapes, paper-based records, pigeon holes, photocopiers, dictation machinery, message books, answer machines etc. Not only the archived material but also the entire 'safe-haven' should be kept locked when not supervised.

4   *Staff access to information in their work*
All members of staff should only be allowed access to confidential information according to their determined level of access.[3] This level of access is determined by the 'data owner' according to the requirements/responsibilities of the job and should be reviewed on a regular basis (*see* Section 9, Information/data 'ownership' and Section 18, Access controls).

The number of staff with access to confidential information should be kept to a minimum.

5   *The procedures for the handling of information*
The Data Protection Act 1998 is the law governing procedures about the handling of confidential information (*see* Chapter 2) and guidelines are given by the Caldicott Principles. It is therefore imperative that every member of staff is familiar with the Data Protection Act 1998 and the Caldicott Principles, which should be a part of staff induction procedures and staff appraisals.

To reduce the possibility of breaches in confidentiality the movements of confidential information outside the physical boundaries of a 'safe haven' should be kept to a minimum. Where possible, multiplication (e.g. photocopy) of confidential information should be avoided.

6   *The receiving of information*
   a   Post: All mail containing patient information should be collected at one entry point within the physical boundaries of a 'safe-haven' to ensure maximum confidentiality. Any mail where it is unclear if patient information is part of its content should be treated as if it would have confidential information.
   b   Fax: Faxes should be placed within the physical boundaries of a 'safe haven' and/or at the very least should be locked when unattended. The policy on the use of fax machines (*see* Section 2, Staff code of conduct) provides guidance on the handling and sending of facsimiles containing patient-identifiable information.
   c   Telephone: Each practice should have a protocol as to which information may be received or given out over the telephone. Information transmitted by telephone should be recorded and handled securely. The identity of the

other party on the telephone must to be confirmed prior to giving out information (*see* also Section 2, Staff code of conduct).

d   Electronic mail: All security procedures also apply to emails (*see* also Section 2).

7   *The disclosure of information*

The disclosure of any confidential information should only be on a need-to-know basis and must adhere to the implied consent of its original disclosure,[4,5] unless disclosure is justified without consent[6] (*see* also disclosure policy in Section 2). Procedures should be established to audit movements of confidential information ('information flow') with the aim of preventing breaches or possible breaches of confidentiality (*see* Section 8, Reviewing information flows).

8   *The storage of information*

Confidential information (independent of the form it has been stored on, i.e. via paper, computer, CCTV images etc.) should be stored in a secure and locked space to which access is controlled and should not be retained any longer than is necessary or required in order to comply with statutory requirements.[7,8] Recorded CCTV images should not be kept for longer than seven days, unless special circumstances apply.[9]

9   *The archiving and destroying of information*

Archived confidential information (independent of its form, i.e. on paper, computer) should be kept locked and access to it should be restricted to authorised persons only.[3]

For guidance on the destroying of information[10,11] please refer to the following information on a records management policy for general practice and to Section 12, Security policy.

10 *The use of computer systems*

Any computer system containing confidential information should have strict access control. It should be protected physically and password controlled.[3] Instructions for using computer programs containing confidential information should also be protected from unauthorised access (*see* Section 18, Access controls).

To achieve compliance with the requirements of Caldicott and data protection a PHCT should have a documented and, with the PCO, agreed policy on records retention and information quality.[12] The following policy on records management, which incorporates both policies, may be printed from www.radcliffe-oxford.com/informationgov on your practice's letter-headed paper and distributed to all members of staff. You may wish to alter this policy to your specific needs. In doing so please ensure that your records management policy meets the necessary local and national requirements. In any circumstances your records management policy should be agreed on by the Caldicott Guardian of your PCO.

Records management policy

The records management policy for general practice will give members of staff guidance on the management of records. The lead responsible for this policy is [name] [job title], who will be in charge of implementing this policy, monitor the compliance with this policy and oversee the training needs of members of staff.

It is the duty of the entire PHCT to maintain an effective records management system and every member of staff must ensure that

- the records are handled according to all legal requirements
- the content of the record is correct and of high quality
- the information is secured
- the access to the records is controlled
- the records are readily accessible and available for use
- the records are properly archived and retained for a specified period of time, but no longer than necessary, and
- the records are properly disposed of or destroyed.

This policy is developed with reference to

- the common law duty of confidence
- the Data Protection Act 1998
- *For the Record*, HSC 1999/053, http://www.doh.gov.uk/ipu
- *Preservation, Retention and Destruction of GP General and Medical Services Records Relating to Patients*, HSC 1998/217, http://www.doh.gov.uk/ipu
- the Public Records Act 1958.

Definition of records

A record is defined in HSC 1999/053 *For the Record* as anything that contains information, in any media (for example paper, electronic such as CDs and floppy disks, images such as photographs, videos or slides, audio tapes), which has been created or gathered as a result of any aspect of the work of NHS employees (which includes agency and casual staff, contractors). The definition of record does not define its content; therefore it does not just relate to patient records but also to records concerning the business, for example administrative records (estates, finances, budgets), audit trials, working papers.

Handling of records

All records should be handled in a way that the information within them

- is of high quality in content and according to the storage medium properly preserved
- is secured, and access secured and controlled according to the sensitivity of the data
- is available to the person who needs it for maximal efficiency, i.e. when and where this person needs it
- is kept for a period of time which is specified by its content.

Data quality of records

The value of a record is determined by its content and therefore it is imperative to have high quality information in the patient records.[13] PRIMIS[14] and GPRD[15] defined standards and procedures for improving data quality in primary care and it is therefore important to visit their websites when developing your own policy on data quality.

Every member of the PHCT has to make certain that according to the remit of his/her job the patient record is

1   *Complete*, i.e. every morbidity of the patient must be recorded.

    a   Every healthcare professional who diagnoses a specific morbidity must ensure that it is coded in the patient's record.

    b   All diagnoses in correspondence about patients are appropriately coded in the patient's record.

    c   The person who issues medication to the patient must ensure that the associated diagnosis is coded.

    d   The person who enters or receives clinical findings (for example: examinations, laboratory tests, x-rays) must check that if there is an associated diagnosis it is coded into the patient's record.

    e   Every healthcare professional who has an encounter with a patient must enter the relevant information into the patient's record.

2   *Accurate*, i.e. the patient's record should be precise.

    a   There should be no inconsistencies in the patient's record

        • the diagnosis should be compatible with the medication issued and
        • the clinical findings are compatible with the recorded diagnosis and
        • there is no evidence of a discrepancy in the patient's record.

        If inconsistencies are found, they must be rectified immediately by the appropriate member of staff.

    b   All the entries must be dated, timed, signed and can be allocated to the person who made the entry. This applies also to all alterations and additions.

    c   All entries must be clear and unambiguous and easy to understand.

    d   The patient should be involved in the data entry as much as possible.

3   *Relevant*: Any entry into the patient record made by a PHCT member of staff should be important. The entry is relevant if the data is in relation to

    a   medical issues

    b   social issues in relation to the patient's care or treatment

    c   legal issues or

    d   insurance purposes

and does not contain jargon, irrelevant speculation, unnecessary abbreviations, non-professional judgements or gossip.

4   *Accessible*: Every healthcare professional who is authorised to use the patient's record should be able to get hold of the information.

    a   The data should be easy to retrieve, for example by a clear filing system.

    b   The data should be held in an appropriate format

        • the handwriting or print must be legible
        • the abbreviations used must be well known.

5 Timely, this means that according to the remit of the job, every PHCT member

   a   should enter patient data into the record as soon as the information becomes available

   b   should ensure that correspondence and results of investigations are merged with the records as soon as possible

   c   should ensure that medical and prescription data are correctly recognised as current or past.

The PHCT has nominated [name] to lead on data quality. [Name] will ensure regular auditing of data quality and ensure that appropriate training takes place.

Retention of records

The Health Service Circular 1998/217 *Preservation, Retention and Destruction of GP General Medical Services Records Relating to Patients* gives guidance on the minimum retention periods for GP medical records.

Record	*Retention period*
• Maternity records	25 years
• Records relating to children and young people (incl paediatric, vaccination, community child health service records)	Until the patient's 25th birthday or 26th if an entry was made when the young person was 17, or 10 years after the death of the patient if sooner
• Records relating to persons receiving treatment for a mental disorder within the meaning of the Mental Health Act 1983	20 years after no further treatment considered necessary or 10 years after the patient's death if sooner
• Records relating to those serving in HM Armed Forces	Not to be destroyed
• Records relating to those serving a prison sentence	Not to be destroyed
• All other personal health records	10 years after the conclusion of treatment

The time period is calculated from the end of the calendar or accounting year following the last entry in the record.

The Fourth Principle of the Data Protection Act 1998 demands that personal data processed for any purpose or purposes shall not be kept for longer than necessary for that purpose or those purposes. The NHS interpretation of this principle is that the retention periods specified in the relevant circulars are the 'necessary' time periods. This means that after the 'necessary' time period the record should be destroyed, unless the reason to keep the record for a longer period of time is otherwise justified. This must be documented carefully as it might constitute a breach of the Data Protection Act and a review period should be set.

Storage of records

Records must always be kept securely when stored, for example in lockable filing cabinets and rooms, and alarmed when the premises is unattended. Besides providing security from unauthorised access the records must also be protected against environmental hazards such as fire and flood.

If records are taken off the premises it is essential to have a comprehensive tracking system that ensures the records can be located quickly and efficiently. The tracking system must ensure that it is clear

* which item has been taken
* who has taken the item and the insurance that this person guarantees its security
* the date of the transfer
* that a receipt has been issued when records are disposed of and returned.

Disposal of records

A record may be disposed of in several different ways, for example by transferring its content from one medium to another (e.g. paper record to electronic records, scanning of letters) or by transferring the record from the PHCT to another organisation, for example for the purpose of archiving.

Before the record is disposed of, the confidentiality of the content of the record has to be ensured at any time during such an action. Transportation arrangements have to comply with the guidance issued by the Information Commissioner, NHS Information Policy Unit and the requirements set out in BS 7799. When using another organisation to archive records it is essential that

* this organisation is registered under the Information Commissioner
* a contract is in place detailing how the records are archived
* the records remain secured and access controlled
* transportation is specified in accordance with guidance and secured
* access is possible without undue delay and a tracker system is established.

Destruction of records

Most NHS records contain sensitive and confidential information and therefore their destruction must be

* undertaken in a secure location
* conducted in a manner that is secure from accident, loss or disclosure
* fully effective, i.e. irreversible either by crosscut-shredding, pulping, incineration or complete mechanical destruction of computer hard disks.

If the destruction cannot be undertaken on site, an approved contractor may take on this task. In this case there should be a formal contract between the practice or PCO and the contractor or supplier. The contract should detail security and confidentiality requirements which include both the transportation and the destruction of the confidential material. A proof of the destruction in the form of a certificate should be obtained. The practice should keep a register of the destruction.

Security incidents and monitoring of compliance

Every member of staff is obliged to report any potential or actual incident (*see* Section 15, Security incidents) if it occurs which should be logged and brought to the attention of the practice Caldicott Guardian.

The practice's Caldicott Guardian will ensure the compliance of the PHCT with this policy.

References

1 DoH (1999) *Protecting and Using Patient Information: a manual for Caldicott Guardians. Controlling access*, March.
2 EL(92)60 issued in 1992: *Handling Confidential Patient Information in Contracting: a code of practice.*
3 Seventh Principle of the Data Protection Act 1998.
4 First Principle of the Data Protection Act 1998.
5 DoH (2003) *Confidentiality: NHS Code of Practice*, version 3.0. http://www.doh.gov.uk/ipu/confiden
6 For example: sections 29, 31(2)(a)(iii), 31(4)(iii), 35 of the Data Protection Act 1998; section 60 of the Health and Social Care Act 2001.
7 HSC 1998/217: *Preservation, Retention and Destruction of GP General and Medical Services Records Relating to Patients.* This Health Service Circular gives guidance on GP records and general record keeping specifying the minimum retention period for GP patient records and where they should be retained.
8 Fifth Principle of the Data Protection Act 1998.
9 Section 51(3)(b) of the Data Protection Act 1998.
10 HSC 1998/217: *Preservation, Retention and Destruction of GP General and Medical Services Records Relating to Patients.* http://www.doh.gov.uk/ipu. This Health Service Circular also provides guidance on the destruction of GP records, when no longer required.
11 HSC 1999/053: *For the Record: managing records in NHS trusts and health authorities.* http://www.doh.gov.uk/ipu
12 http://nww.nhsia.nhs.uk/infogov/igt/RequirementsList
13 Third and Fourth Principle of the Data Protection Act 1998.
14 PRIMIS (Primary Care Information Services) facilitator's handbook: http://www.primis.nhs.uk/.
15 GPRD (General Practice Research Database): http://www.gprd.com/.

Section 11
Protocols to govern information sharing

Protocols governing information sharing have to be drawn-up.[1–3] As this will need time to be developed, the following will outline the principles of and provide guidance for what should be achieved through these protocols. At a later time the PCT/PCO will be a signatory to any local protocols governing the disclosure or exchange of patient information with other organisations (social services, police [Crime and Disorder Act 1998], education services, voluntary sector providers, private sector providers).

Every transfer of confidential information should be governed by clear and transparent protocols that satisfy the requirements of the law. The information should only be used for agreed on and legitimate purposes, and only disclosed on a need-to-know basis to achieve seamless care.[4]

Until these protocols are developed, each PHCT should adapt the following principles when 'sharing'/passing on information:

- Those concerned with the care of a patient/client should have ready access to the information needed, keeping it confidential and respecting privacy.
- The obligation to safeguard confidential information should be governed (besides by the law) by contracts of employment and professional codes of conduct.[5]
- As long as the individual is working within the defined protocol there will be no need to gain specific consent each time information is passed on.
- Access to information should only be granted on a strict need-to-know basis.
- An individual's wishes should be respected unless exceptional circumstances (e.g. statute or court order, public health risk, harm to other individuals, or the prevention, detection or prosecution of serious crime) prevail.[6]
- Where information on individuals has been aggregated or anonymised, it should still be used for justified purposes only.[4]
- The receiving organisation is to meet agreed standards, e.g.:[5]

  - information should only be accessed by those involved in the care of patients on a need-to-know basis
  - mechanisms should be in place to ensure physical security (e.g. locked storage cabinets, security protected computer systems), security awareness and training, in security management, system development, and security policies
  - besides the physical security of IT the data contained within it should be secured as well
  - all information should be password protected.

References

1   HSC 1999/012: *Caldicott Guardians*.
2   DoH (1999) *Protecting and Using Patient Information: a manual for Caldicott Guardians. Protocols governing the receipt and disclosure of patient/client information*, March.

3 DoH (2003) *Confidentiality: NHS Code of Practice*, version 3.0. http://www. doh.gov.uk/ipu/confiden

4 First, Second and Third Principle of the Data Protection Act 1998.

5 Seventh Principle of the Data Protection Act 1998.

6 First Principle of the Data Protection Act 1998.

Section 12
Security policy

(You might like to print this security policy from www.radcliffe-oxford.com/informationgov.)

Introduction

It is a necessity for every practice to develop a security policy to protect all information-processing systems in healthcare adequately.[1–4] The increasing reliance on IT which aims to improve the efficiency and effectiveness of the delivery of care makes it necessary that information systems are safe, secure, operational and properly used and maintained. This includes not only electronic systems but also paper-based information, images (including CCTV)[5] and verbal records.

To achieve this, the security policy should set out guidelines and protocols that ensure the physical, procedural and logical security and regulate the management, distribution and protection of data/materials.[6,7]

The NHS has adopted the BS 7799 national standard for security.[8] This code of practice contains a wide range of information security, management policies and practices.

The most important UK Acts that cover some aspects of information security are:

- Data Protection Act 1998
- Access to Health Records Act 1990
- Computer Misuse Act 1990
- Human Rights Act 1998
- Freedom of Information Act 2000
- The Copyright, Designs and Patents Act 1988.

Scope of security policy

- The aim of this and the following sections is to ensure that information processing is properly assessed for security.
- By developing proper levels of security the confidentiality as well as the integrity and availability of information are achieved.
- Every member of staff should be aware of his/her role, accountability and responsibilities.
- Through audit and incident reporting the awareness of information security issues is raised and security needs and systems are improved.

Information security

The security of information will be achieved by guaranteeing that the following three components are fulfilled:

- Confidentiality: Information can be only accessed by those who have got the authority, on a need-to-know basis.

- Integrity: All components of the system are operating correctly and according to specification and all information is suitable for the purpose for which it was collected.
- Availability: Information is comprehensively accessible whenever it is needed (but only to those who are authorised).

The contents of security policy

This section, 'Security policy', should be read in connection with the following sections:

- Security responsibilities (Section 13)
- Risk assessment and management (Section 14)
- Security incidents and monitoring (Sections 15 and 16)
- User responsibilities (Section 17)
- Access controls (Section 18).

Together these form a comprehensive information security policy.

The following topics will be covered in this section:

1   equipment security
2   maintenance of the equipment
3   maintaining the confidentiality of all data within the practice
4   the disposal of confidential material or equipment containing confidential information
5   protocol regarding the use and maintenance of CCTV equipment.

Equipment security

- IM&T equipment should be installed and used according to the manufacturer's specification.
- Physical access to confidential material should be restricted in order to avoid un-authorised access, i.e. windows and doors should be secured when unattended.
- The same strict security measures should be in place for any portable data machines.
- Site computers and printers and fax machines should be kept away from public view or windows.
- Protection against damage or interruption to its use/function should be en-sured through proper power supplies and proper cabling as well as protection against environmental hazards such as damp/flood, spillage, overheating/fire, dust/smoke etc.
- A tested protocol for 'disaster recovery' (i.e. how data are to be retrieved or made accessible) should be in place.
- All equipment should be logged with serial numbers so it can be easily identified.
- All equipment should be security marked.
- Conservation of equipment:

– Maintenance agreements should be arranged according to the manufacturer's specification.
– Only approved systems engineers should be contracted for maintenance and allowed to have access to hardware or software.
– If during repairs/maintenance engineers could gain access to confidential materials they should sign a confidentiality agreement and a member of staff should be present during the maintenance and repair operation.
– A record of faults or suspected faults should be maintained.
– Backups:

  ○ have a documented procedure for the daily backup
  ○ store off site or in a fireproof safe and secured from physical loss
  ○ test the backup procedure regularly
  ○ as a minimal requirement have a three-tape system so that even if the backup procedures fail only a small amount of data is lost.

– Virus protection:

  ○ users should report any detected or suspected viruses immediately
  ○ anti-virus software should be updated regularly
  ○ PC should be checked regularly for viruses
  ○ the person in charge of security in the practice should be informed and has to agree to any new installation of computer software/program
  ○ any new sets of data, disks, software should be virus checked prior to their use
  ○ computer games should not be installed on computers and staff should be warned about free disks from magazines, 'pirate' software, programs from 'bulletin boards'
  ○ adequate backup procedures should be established.

– In the event of a virus infection:

  ○ notify the line manager as soon as a virus is detected
  ○ isolate infected machine immediately
  ○ check all possibly infected machines for the virus – and if in doubt isolate machine(s)
  ○ prevent the re-use of the infected machine until its safety has been approved
  ○ infected machine: memory and disk should be wiped clean, the master copy of software reloaded, data from most recent backups should be reloaded.

Maintenance of the equipment

• Repairing or servicing of computer systems by external contractors must be subject to confidentiality agreements.
• Staff have to learn how the system should be used and kept up to date with changes which may affect functionality.
• Care has to be taken when computers or software programs are to be disposed of. The memory (e.g. on hard disk) has to be deleted before disposal to ensure that patient-identifiable information can not be retrieved.

- When purchasing and installing any new system or new software the security implications should be actively considered; also a check for viruses before use is required.
- Make sure that clinical records are kept up to date.

Maintaining the confidentiality of all data within the practice

- Ensure that only authorised persons can gain access to your computer system (*see* Section 18, Access controls).
- Do not disclose any information to anyone who does not have the right to see it and pass on patient information on a need-to-know basis only.
- Access to the computer should be secured by passwords.
- 'Exit'/log-off the system whenever you are leaving your screen unattended, so that the next person needs to log into the system with his/her password to work with the computer.
- Ensure that all equipment is protected from intruders.
- Virus-check all disks and software coming into the practice.

The disposal of confidential material or equipment containing confidential information

- Only after consultation with the appropriate healthcare professional should health records be destroyed; guidance for the retention periods for GP medical records is given in HSC 1998/217[9] and HSC 1999/053[10] (*see* also records management policy in Section 10, Safe-haven procedures).
- Ensuring that confidentiality is maintained throughout the process of destruction of confidential patient/staff records must be the highest priority.
- The disposal of any storage media such as computers/hard disks, diskettes, magnetic/DAT tapes, films, and also ink ribbons for fax machines should only take place after the data contained on it have been reliably destroyed.
- Paper records should be crosscut-shredded or incinerated.
- Floppy disks should be cut because deleting data or formatting are reversible procedures.
- Hard drives should be drilled to be destroyed.
- The destruction procedure should be documented by the person who is in charge of confidentiality and security in the practice.
- A contractor who has government approval for the destruction of confidential waste should be used unless the PHCT disposes of confidential items on its own.

Protocol regarding the use and maintenance of CCTV equipment[11]

- A designated member of staff should be in charge of the following security policy for CCTV and monitor the compliance of members of staff with this security policy (*see* also Chapter 2).

- The CCTV equipment should be positioned appropriately to achieve its purpose for crime protection and public safety, i.e. camera(s) are located to observe only the area intended for surveillance and monitor(s) positioned so they can be overlooked by designated staff.
- The CCTV equipment should function properly, tapes should be of good quality, replaced on a regular basis to guarantee clear images and images produced with reference to location of camera and date and time.
- The equipment should be maintained and serviced according to specifications: ensuring the upkeep, cleaning, timely repair and replacement of faulty equipment, and documented in an up-to-date log-book.
- Location of the equipment should also be chosen in view of minimising the possibility of vandalism or physical interference.
- Recorded images should be kept safe, locked up and not kept longer than necessary.
- As soon as the images are not required any more (normally about seven days unless special circumstances apply) they should be removed or erased.
- Access to the images should be controlled for authorised members of staff only and be documented (*see* Section 18, Access controls).

References

1   DoH (1999) *Protecting and Using Patient Information: a manual for Caldicott Guardians. Management audits and improvement plans*, March.
2   NHS Executive's Security and Data Protection Programme (1999) *Play IT Safe: a practical guide to IT security for everyone working in general practice*, version 1.1. Available from the NHS Information Authority.
3   NHS Executive's Security and Data Protection Programme (1999) *Ensuring Security and Confidentiality in NHS Organisations: protecting the security of information in NHS organisations*, IMG Ref No E5501.
4   Seventh Principle of the Data Protection Act.
5   Section 51(3)(b) of the Data Protection Act 1998. *See* also NHS Executive (1996) *Guidance on Video Recording NHS Operations*, issued under cover of a letter from the chief executive.
6   NHS Executive's Security and Data Protection Programme (1999) *The Handbook of Information Security: information security in general practice*. Available from the NHS Information Authority.
7   Dr Ross J Anderson (1996) *Security in Clinical Information Systems*, January. Consultation paper commissioned for the BMA Council by the BMA Information Technology Committee.
8   BS 7799-1:1999: *Information Security Management – Part 1: Code of practice for information security management*. http://www.nhsia.nhs.uk/erdip/pages/docs_egif/evaluation/technical/ehr-req-final.pdf
9   HSC 1998/217. This Health Service Circular gives guidance on GP medical records. The Information Policy Unit at the DoH publishes regular advice on information security on the IPU website at http://www.doh.gov.uk/ipu. Update No 2 July 2002 gives their advice on data destruction.

10 HSC 1999/053: *For the Record: managing records in NHS trusts and health authorities*. This circular lists suggestions of minimum periods for retention of NHS records. HSC 1998/217 specifically covers GP medical records and is therefore more relevant to general practice; HSC 1999/053 is about the management of GP records held by health authorities and NHS trusts.

11 Section 51(3)(b) of the Data Protection Act 1998.

Section 13
Security responsibilities

'Security responsibilities' is an element of a comprehensive security policy (*see* Section 12, Security policy).[1,2] The PHCT has a legal obligation to ensure the confidentiality and security of all confidential materials at all times.[3] Therefore the practice's Caldicott Guardian/Information Governance Lead or the GP who is in overall charge of maintaining and ensuring confidentiality of all confidential material/data in the practice has the following responsibilities (you might like to print these responsibilities from www.radcliffe-oxford.com/informationgov on your practice's letter-headed paper).

- Making it clear and obvious – from inside the PHCT and from the outside – who is in charge of the security of IM&T. This may be the practice's Caldicott Guardian or the GP himself or herself.
- Ensuring that the person in charge of IM&T has had sufficient training that guarantees an adequate standard of ability to fulfil his/her role as a leader on IM&T security.
- The person in charge of IM&T security will need to achieve the following objectives:
  - ensuring the implementation of security policy (*see* Section 12) and other policies/guidelines, e.g. safe-haven procedures (*see* Section 10)
  - ensuring compliance with the Data Protection Act (*see* Chapter 2), common law duty of confidentiality and other relevant legislation as well as with Caldicott requirements
  - making sure that staff are aware of their responsibilities
  - making sure that employees have signed a written statement as to their responsibilities concerning the security of confidential material/data
  - raising awareness e.g. by setting up regular meetings to discuss matters of security and confidentiality within the practice
  - ensuring that arrangements are in place for the disposal of confidential material/data, e.g. paper, old computers (*see* Section 12, Security policy)
  - making sure that there are adequate backup procedures in place and adequate storage provided
  - making sure that no vital equipment or software is taken from the premises
  - ensuring that it is clear who has the ownership of which confidential material including the responsibilities that ownership confers (*see* Section 9, Information/data 'ownership')
  - maintaining a record of all actual and potential security breaches
  - performing audits and initiating improvements (*see* Section 16, Security monitoring)
  - ensuring that every member of staff has his/her training needs assessed, staff receive their training and a record of all training sessions is kept (*see* Section 4, Confidentiality and security training needs)
  - controlling the access to confidential material (*see* Section 18, Access controls).
- Making sure that all members of staff using IM&T support the person in charge of IM&T security.

References

1 BS 7799-1:1999: *Information Security Management – Part 1: Code of practice for information security management.* http://www.nhsia.nhs.uk/erdip/pages/docs_egif/evaluation/technical/ehr-req-final.pdf

2 NHS Executive's Security and Data Protection Programme (1999) *Ensuring Security and Confidentiality in NHS Organisations: protecting the security of information in NHS organisations,* IMG Ref No E5501.

3 Seventh Principle of the Data Protection Act.

Section 14
Risk assessment and management

'Risk assessment and management' is also an important element of a complete security policy (*see* Section 12).[1,2] In order to have or introduce effective security measures to safeguard confidential information a risk assessment should be performed.[3] This should be performed on a regular basis (annually) as localities, inventories and information processing change continually. The risk assessment should be executed by following the CCTA Risk Analysis and Management Method (CRAMM), though a full CRAMM study will not always be necessary.

All data and equipment should be assessed for the possibility of a security threat, and the severity of damage if such a security threat would occur to sensitive information (i.e. any patient-identifiable information).[4]

A risk assessment consists of four components: the inventory, the possibility of a security threat, the possible resulting impact and the vulnerability.

1   The inventory of equipment. The value/importance of equipment is measured by the impact a loss/destruction would cause (e.g. personal distress, legal fines, bad publicity/embarrassment):

   a   paper records/files/letters/incoming or outgoing post
   b   computer hardware and software, printers
   c   backup tapes
   d   fax machines/answerphones.

2   The assessment of the possibility of a security threat, which includes:

   a   physical damage (fire, flood, vandalism)
   b   theft
   c   unauthorised/adverse (virus/program failure), modification
   d   unauthorised disclosure.

3   The assessment of the possible impact of any security threat with regard to the risk to the individual patients and the practice (e.g. disclosure of data, destruction of data/equipment/software, unauthorised or incorrect modification of data).
   The assessment should take into account:

   a   which type of information and
   b   the degree of severity of a possible security threat.

4   Vulnerability is the weakness or liability in the system or its environment that may be exploited in the occurrence of a threat. In order to measure the vulnerability an assessment of the probability that a threat will succeed in causing harm of damage is needed (e.g. unlocked doors, open windows, written down passwords).

Scoring system

To facilitate the assessment a scoring system has been developed. It should help to identify areas of high risks and to prioritise the introduction of preventive measures.

Possibility of threat:	Rare	1
	Unlikely	2
	Possible	3
	Likely	4
	Definite	5
Possible implication:	Negligible	1
	Low	2
	Medium	3
	Very high	4
	Extreme	5
Vulnerability:	None	1
	Little effect	2
	Moderate effect	3
	High effect	4

To perform a risk analysis each item of the material/data should be ascribed an estimated degree (as above) for the risk of a threat, its vulnerability and impact. Then take the mathematical product, i.e.

$$\text{Threat} \times \text{Vulnerability} \times \text{Impact} = \text{Risk}$$

This risk analysis not only gives guidance for prioritising efforts to reduce the risk but also an indication of how best to reduce the risk, i.e. either improve security in order to reduce the threat or reduce the vulnerability by taking measures against the threat.

The following is a guide as to how such an assessment could be set up. It is a basic risk assessment tool for physical items and modifications for the individual surgery will need to be made.

A similar layout can be used to assess other risks such as 'logical' security risks, e.g.:

- access: password use, screen savers (*see* Section 18, Access controls)
- backup systems in place (*see* Section 12, Security policy)
- disposal of data (*see* Section 12)
- virus protection (*see* Section 12).

General practice – risk assessment

Name of assessor: _____

Date of assessment: ___/___/___

Assessment item	Threat	Vulnerability	Impact	Score	Action plan
Computers:					
Reception area Serial No.					
Treatment room Serial No.					
Consultation room 1 Serial No.					
Consultation room 2 Serial No.					
Secretary Serial No.					
Practice manager Serial No.					
Computer software					
Dictaphone tapes					
Backup tapes					
Paper records					
Letters					
Lab reports					
Scripts (for collection)					
Fax machines					
Message book					
Visit book					
Pigeon holes					

Signed by assessor: _____   Date: ___/___/___

References

1 BS 7799-1:1999: *Information Security Management – Part 1: Code of practice for information security management.* http://www.nhsia.nhs.uk/erdip/pages/docs_egif/evaluation/technical/ehr-req-final.pdf

2 NHS Executive's Security and Data Protection Programme (1999) *Ensuring Security and Confidentiality in NHS Organisations: protecting the security of information in NHS organisations,* IMG Ref No E5501.

3 Seventh Principle of the Data Protection Act 1998.

4 NHS Executive's Security and Data Protection Programme (1999) *The Handbook of Information Security: information security in general practice.* Available from the NHS Information Authority.

Section 15
Security incidents

'Security incidents' is another important element of a good and wide-ranging security policy (*see* Section 12).[1]

Security of information

Security of information is achieved by ensuring that the following three components are guaranteed (*see* Section 12, Security policy).[2,3]

1 *Confidentiality*: Information is only accessed by those who have the authority and on a need-to-know basis.
2 *Integrity*: All systems are operating correctly and according to specifications and all information is suitable for the purpose for which it was collected.
3 *Availability*: Information is comprehensively accessible whenever needed (but only to those who are authorised).

Types of security incidents

A security incident is defined as any event that resulted or had the potential to result in a violation of any of the three components above, i.e.:

- *information has been disclosed to an unauthorised person* because of e.g. inadequate disposal of confidential material, the use of a wrong password, an intruder on the premises
- *the integrity of the system or its information has been put at risk* because of e.g. theft or damage of computers, dictaphones, unauthorised and inappropriate modification of information
- *the availability of the system or information has been put at risk* because of e.g. power failure, failure to have backup tapes.

Classification of incident severity

The severity of the impact depends upon the adverse impact the incident might have, i.e. the risk of

- harm to the patient's safety or confidentiality/privacy and integrity
- a penalty or the lack of the fulfilment of legal obligations
- an economic impact
- embarrassment to the profession or healthcare provider.

  1 defines high risk
  2 defines intermediate risk
  3 defines low risk.

Security incidents reporting

All actual or possible security incidents must be reported, even if they have been innocently or unintentionally caused. Every member of staff should know to whom such reports should be made within the PHCT (practice's Caldicott Guardian/practice manager/GP).

High-risk security incidents that involve IT system security or NHSnet should also be reported to the Caldicott Guardian or Clinical Governance Lead in the PCO/PCT. It is imperative to ensure absolute protection and confidentiality for the reporting party.

A report on a security incident should at least contain the following items:

- the person(s) involved
- the date
- the location
- the type/description of the incident.

The following gives guidance on how to deal with a security incident and an example of a security incident report form. You might like to print the security incident report form from www.radcliffe-oxford.com/informationgov.

Guidance on dealing with a security incident

- One person in the practice – e.g. GP, practice's Caldicott Guardian, practice manager – should be nominated to follow up security incidents and keep a log-book.
- A security incident should be classified as high, intermediate or low risk.
- Its impact should be considered, e.g. do patients need to be informed of the leak of confidential information, is the virus threatening other computers, and so on.
- If any criminal activity has occurred (theft, vandalism) the police should be involved.
- Consider if others need to be informed, e.g. system suppliers, IM&T lead or Caldicott Guardian and/or the Clinical Governance Lead in the PCO/PCT.
- Investigate if existing policies or guidelines have been adhered to by staff involved in the incident.
- Consider if there are any weaknesses in the existing policies or guidelines.
- Consider how future security incidents of this sort can be avoided, e.g. by amending existing policies or guidelines, better staff training, improved security (alarm systems).
- New policies and guidelines should be handed out to every member of staff.

Security incident report

Name:
(reporting the incident)

Person(s) involved:

Location of incident:

Date of incident: /   /

Report of actual/possible security incident:

Signed: _____   Date: /   /

For management use only:

Risk classification: high
                          intermediate
                          low

Action taken/required:

Security incident reported to:

Signed: _____   Date: /   /
(Practice's Caldicott Guardian/practice manager/GP)

References

1   NHS Executive's Security and Data Protection Programme (1999) *The Handbook of Information Security: information security in general practice.* Available from the NHS Information Authority.

2   BS 7799-1:1999: *Information Security Management – Part 1: Code of practice for information security management.* http://www.nhsia.nhs.uk/erdip/pages/docs_egif/evaluation/technical/ehr-req-final.pdf

3   NHS Executive's Security and Data Protection Programme (1999) *Ensuring Security and Confidentiality in NHS Organisations: protecting the security of information in NHS organisations,* IMG Ref No E5501.

Section 16
Security monitoring

'Security monitoring' is a further necessary element of a comprehensive security policy (*see* Section 12) and has an important function in improving the effectiveness of security measures and raising awareness of staff members on security matters.[1,2] Security monitoring should therefore involve the entire PHCT and should take place on a regular basis.

Security monitoring should include:

*   reviewing potential or actual security breaches, and if necessary developing an action plan to improve security
*   audits which review the compliance with the guidance on any aspect of security, e.g. access failures, log-on/log-off procedures, password usage, safe-haven procedures, information flow, compliance with the Data Protection Act 1998 etc.

The results of such reviews and the resulting changes in security measures or changes to guidelines and protocols should be documented in a report and kept for an agreed period of time as well as handed out to all members of the PHCT.

Please file these reports.

Report on audit/security review

Name of practice: _____

Practice address: _____

_____

_____ Postcode: _____

Topic of audit/security review: _____

_____

_____

_____

Findings of audit/security review: _____

_____

_____

_____

_____

_____

_____

_____

Resulting action plan: _____

_____

_____

_____

_____

Signature: _____ Date: ___ / ___ / ___

(Practice's Caldicott Guardian/practice manager/GP)

References

1   BS 7799-1:1999: *Information Security Management – Part 1: Code of practice for information security management.* http://www.nhsia.nhs.uk/erdip/pages/docs_egif/evaluation/technical/ehr-req-final.pdf

2   NHS Executive's Security and Data Protection Programme (1999) *Ensuring Security and Confidentiality in NHS Organisations: protecting the security of information in NHS organisations,* IMG Ref No E5501.

Section 17
User responsibilities

'User responsibilities' is a further significant issue that a comprehensive security policy should cover (*see* Section 12). This section is aimed especially at the users of IM&T equipment and their need to understand their responsibilities in safeguarding personal data and in the maintenance of equipment.[1–3] Users are members of staff having direct or delegated responsibilities for the entering, retrieval, care and maintenance of personal-identifiable data or information.[4]

Part of a good security policy is that the user knows his/her responsibilities. This can only be achieved through the regular review of training needs and the raising of awareness as well as regular reviews of policies, protocols and guidelines.

Most of the topics of this section have already been covered in this book and therefore it should be read in connection with these sections, especially those covering security policy (Section 12) and staff code of conduct (Section 2) in this chapter.

The main aspects of user responsibilities are the following:

- To maintain confidentiality and to ensure availability of information within the responsibilities of the job.
- To ensure that all physical security measures are properly used.
- Rules regarding passwords should be observed (*see* Section 18, Access controls).
- Clear desk, clear screen policy:

  - after each consultation/session all sensitive information should be removed from view before starting the next consultation/session
  - reception areas should be clear of any sensitive information which should be out of sight and out of reach of any unauthorised person
  - 'sensitive areas' (such as consultation rooms or offices) should be locked when not in use
  - the user of a computer should log-off prior to leaving the room
  - there should be an automatic activation of screen savers after a certain period of time
  - screen savers should be password protected for reactivation
  - computer screens and printers should be out of view of any unauthorised person.

- Computer users have to make sure that no potential or actual security breaches occur as a result of their action.
- Any storage media (e.g. disks, tapes) which contain patient-identifiable information should be stored in a locked, fireproof safe.
- Records should be kept up to date.
- Software should only be loaded onto the computer after authorisation by the practice's Caldicott Guardian/practice manager or GP and after it has been checked for viruses.
- Disks should also be checked for viruses before they are loaded on the computer.
- All computer records and printouts should be disposed of confidentially either via crosscut-shredding, incineration or sent for disposal with other confidential waste.

- Access should only be granted on a need-to-know basis.
- Incidents of security breaches, faults of equipment or any other irregularities should be reported (*see* Section 15, Security incidents).
- Intruders should be challenged.
- A written statement should be signed concerning the responsibilities they have taken on in regard to the security of confidential material and data.
- To ensure that the information gained during the course of employment remains confidential after the termination of employment (*see* Section 6, Staff contracts).
- The Data Protection Act 1998, Caldicott Principles and all relevant legislation should be complied with.
- Users of CCTV equipment should be trained in the recognition and application of privacy rights and their implication with regard to recorded images (*see* also Chapter 2).[5]

References

1   NHS Executive's Security and Data Protection Programme (1999) *Play IT Safe: a practical guide to IT security for everyone working in general practice*, version 1.1. Available from the NHS Information Authority.

2   BS 7799-1:1999: *Information Security Management – Part 1: Code of practice for information security management.* http://www.nhsia.nhs.uk/erdip/pages/docs_egif/evaluation/technical/ehr-req-final.pdf

3   NHS Executive's Security and Data Protection Programme (1999) *Ensuring Security and Confidentiality in NHS Organisations: protecting the security of information in NHS organisations*, IMG Ref No E5501.

4   Second, Third and Fourth Principle of the Data Protection Act 1998: http://www.hmso.gov.uk/acts/acts1998/19980029.htm and http://www.informationcommissioner.gov.uk.

5   Section 51(3)(b) of the Data Protection Act 1998: http://www.hmso.gov.uk/acts/acts1998/19980029.htm.

Section 18
Access controls

'Access controls' is another element of a comprehensive security policy (*see* Section 12). In order to protect patient confidentiality and privacy it is essential that access to confidential information is controlled, limiting it to authorised persons only.[1] This section offers guidance on how to control physical and logical access to confidential material.[2,3]

Controlled physical access

- All central processors/file servers, and any other confidential material should be located in secure areas with restricted access through a physical barrier.
- Locks on doors, closed windows, computer secured to desks, installed alarms etc.
- Access should be limited to the 'bare necessities'.
- Access to recorded images/CCTV[4] should be restricted to those members of staff who need to have access to achieve its defined purpose (*see* also Chapter 2):

  - all requests to access stored images should be documented
  - any access to stored images should be documented
  - disclosure of recorded images by a third party should be limited to special circumstances
  - prior to disclosure of images, any third party whose image is not to be disclosed should have his/her image disguised or blurred.

- External agencies should not be given access unless formally authorised (*see* Section 7, Contracts placed with other organisations), and should be accompanied throughout the visit.

Controlled logical access
The prevention of misuse

- All computers should be installed with password-protected screen savers, so that there is no risk of unauthorised access if they are left unattended for a short period of time.
- On computer screens giving access to sensitive data, a message should be displayed warning that unauthorised access is a criminal offence.
- Staff should be aware that the Computer Misuse Act 1990 introduced three criminal offences:

  1 unauthorised access
  2 unauthorised access with the intent to commit a further serious offence
  3 unauthorised modification of computer material.

User registration

Access control also requires the determination of who should be allowed access to confidential material/data and to which level.[1] Before giving staff members access to confidential information they should be properly trained and certain principles (*see* Caldicott Principles)[5] should be observed which form the basis for granting access to these confidential material/data.

- The *minimum possible number of staff* should have access to the *minimum necessary confidential data* (i.e. name, address, DoB, patient records, etc.).
- The purpose of the access to confidential data has to be *justified*.
- Access levels have to be granted on a *strict need-to-know* basis.
- Staff who have access to confidential data should *understand the law and comply with it*.
- Staff who have access to confidential/person-identifiable information have to *understand their responsibilities*.
- The 'rights of access' and access levels of staff have to be reviewed periodically.

The final page of this section is a form, which should be completed for each IM&T user in the practice. An initial password should be issued which the user should change to his/her *own* password during the first IM&T session. Written details of access rights and responsibilities should be issued to every user (*see* Section 17, User responsibilities). A record should be kept with the user's personal file.

Guidance on password use

All new users must be briefed on the importance of passwords. The following instructions are essential.

- Always log into the system using *your own* password, i.e. the password should be self-selected, individual, and not known to anyone else.
- Use a password that cannot be easily guessed because it relates to you (e.g. name of your child, dog or favourite cartoon character). Simple rules about passwords are:

  – do not use one letter twice
  – use at least one different character which is not part of the alphabet
  – use at least six symbols (example: 4*SPLMI as an abbreviation of the sentence: For * Sake Please Let Me In).

- You have to keep your password secret. Do *not* share your password or write it down.
- You should only use the computer system *within the remit* of your job. (Newer computer systems have got different access levels for users according to the needs of their jobs. The person in charge of IT in the practice should make sure that staff are receiving access levels on a need-to-know basis.)
- *Change* your user password at *regular intervals* (monthly).
- *Notify* your supervisor of any case of *breach or misuse* of your log-on or any other observed or attempted irregularity.

The person in charge of IT in the practice should make sure when a staff member is leaving the practice that his/her access to the computer system is terminated.

Log-on and log-off procedures

To ensure that only authorised persons can gain access to your IM&T system, access should be controlled via a log-on process, which is designed to minimise unauthorised access. Standards for a secure log-on process are as follows:

- The system should not display any identifiers or help messages until the log-on has been successfully completed.
- If an error occurs during a log-on, the system should not indicate which part of the data was correct or incorrect.
- The number of unsuccessful log-on attempts should be limited to three, after which a record is made and data link connections are disconnected.
- After a successful log-on, a display of the last successful log-on and details of any unsuccessful log-on attempts should appear on the screen.
- Users should log-off terminals/PC when leaving them unattended.
- After a terminal has not been used for a pre-set period of time the screen should clear and the application and network session should close.

Third-party access

A third party should only be allowed to gain access to NHS facilities if contractual arrangements ensure that NHS security requirements are met (*see* Section 7, Contracts placed with other organisations).

It might be necessary to perform a risk assessment and introduce protective measures prior to letting a third party gain access.

Every IM&T user in the PHCT should be registered and complete the following form with the practice's Caldicott Guardian or practice manager or GP. The registration status of every employee should be regularly reviewed. You might like to print this registration form from www.radcliffe-oxford.com/informationgov.

Registration of IM&T system users

Employee's name: _____

Position: _____

Job description: _____

_____

_____

IT access needed for: _____

_____

Access level issued: _____

Date issued: ___ / ___ / ___   Review date: ___ / ___ / ___

Before granting access to the IT system, the employee has been informed about, has understood, and received a copy of the security policy and guidelines on user responsibilities and access controls. The employee has received adequate training in the use of the IT system.

Signature of employee: _____

Authorised by (signature): _____
(Practice's Caldicott Guardian/practice manager/GP)

Modification/De-registration

Reason: _____

Actions taken: _____

_____

_____

_____

_____

Name: _____
(Practice's Caldicott Guardian/practice manager/GP)

Signature: _____ Date: __/__/____
(Practice's Caldicott Guardian/practice manager/GP)

References

1 Seventh Principle of the Data Protection Act 1998.
2 NHS Executive's Security and Data Protection Programme (1999) *Ensuring Security and Confidentiality in NHS Organisations: protecting the security of information in NHS organisations*, IMG Ref No E5501.
3 BS 7799-1:1999: *Information Security Management – Part 1: Code of practice for information security management*. http://www.nhsia.nhs.uk/erdip/pages/docs_egif/evaluation/technical/ehr-req-final.pdf
4 Section 51(3)(b) of the Data Protection Act 1998. *See* also CCTV in Chapter 2.
5 DoH (1997) *The Caldicott Committee Report on the Review of Patient-identifiable Information*, December. http://www.hmso.gov.uk/confiden/app2.htm

Section 19
Information governance assessment

The following audit questionnaire will give the reader a chance to assess his/her practice's performance against the standards set out in the Caldicott Report and the Data Protection Act. This questionnaire should assist in finding areas that are in need of improvement and help to formulate the practice strategy to improve on confidentiality and data protection.

The numbers of each set of questions correspond to the number of each section in this chapter. For further explanation of what is meant by or intended to be covered by a question posed in this questionnaire, the corresponding section in this chapter should provide the help and guidance needed in the understanding of this question.

The NHS Information Authority has published an Information Governance Toolkit (IG Toolkit) with 24 standards on confidentiality code of practice and 19 standards on data protection for general practice.[1] Performing well in the following audit questionnaire will enable you to satisfy easily all the standards set out by the NHS Information Authority IG Toolkit. It will be helpful to become familiar with the IG Toolkit website.

You might want to amend the audit to make it more suitable for your PHCT, but be sure not to miss out on minimal requirements. You might like to print this questionnaire from www.radcliffe-oxford.com/informationgov.

Please tick boxes Yes or No ☑ ☒

1 **Caldicott Guardian/information governance lead**
  a Has your PHCT nominated a person in charge of data
     protection, confidentiality and data security? ☐ ☐
  b Did this person receive adequate training for this role? ☐ ☐
  c Is this person supported by all senior members of
     the PHCT? ☐ ☐
  d Has this person ensured that the practice's data protection
     notification is comprehensive and up to date? ☐ ☐
  e Has this person ensured that all the practice's policies and
     guidelines are in line with national policies and guidance? ☐ ☐

2 **Staff code of conduct**
  a Does a code of conduct in respect of confidentiality exist
     for all your members of staff/employees? ☐ ☐
     Does the code of conduct include:
     i   instructions on how to handle confidential information ☐ ☐
     ii how to deal with confidential information given/
         received over the phone or answering machine ☐ ☐
     iii how to deal with faxes ☐ ☐
     iv a reference to disciplinary procedures in the case of a
         breach of the code of conduct ☐ ☐
     v   when patient information may be disclosed ☐ ☐
     vi how to secure your working space? ☐ ☐
  b Has every member of your PHCT received a code of
     conduct and understood its content? ☐ ☐
  c Is this code of conduct reviewed and updated on a regular
     basis (e.g. due to a change in working patterns, after a
     security incident, or as the result of an audit)? ☐ ☐

3 **Staff induction procedures**
  a Are all new members of staff made aware and given a
     comprehensive and systematic introduction of their duties
     and responsibilities with regards to data protection and
     confidentiality at the commencement of their employment? ☐ ☐
  b Are the new members of staff given a written copy of all
     the relevant practice's policies, e.g.:
     i   staff code of conduct ☐ ☐
     ii principles of Data Protection Act/Caldicott ☐ ☐
     iii practice's security policy ☐ ☐
     iv security responsibility ☐ ☐
     v   safe-haven procedures? ☐ ☐
  c Has the new employee signed a statement that he/she has
     had explained and understands the above policies,
     principles and procedures after they have been discussed
     with him/her? ☐ ☐
  d Has the access level to confidential data been determined? ☐ ☐

4 Confidentiality and security training needs

a   Are the training needs of all members of staff systematically
    assessed, and confidentiality and security issues reinforced?   ☐   ☐
    Have key areas been covered e.g.:
    i   access controls   ☐   ☐
    ii   Caldicott Principles   ☐   ☐
    iii   Data Protection Act   ☐   ☐
    iv   other law/legal requirements   ☐   ☐
    v   IM&T skills   ☐   ☐
    vi   safe-haven procedures   ☐   ☐
    vii   security policy   ☐   ☐
    viii security responsibilities   ☐   ☐
    ix   staff code of conduct   ☐   ☐
    x   user responsibilities   ☐   ☐
    xi   additional practice policies?   ☐   ☐

b   Are training needs adjusted to each individual's needs and
    updated to incorporate changes in working environment,
    or changes in job roles?   ☐   ☐

c   Are the training needs regularly assessed yearly and do they
    form part of a personal development plan or appraisal?   ☐   ☐

5 Communication with patients/information for patients

a   Does your practice have a communication strategy?   ☐   ☐

b   Does your practice have a patient information leaflet?   ☐   ☐
    i   Has your practice got an up-to-date (revised in the
         last 12 months) patient information leaflet?   ☐   ☐
    ii   Does the patient information leaflet inform patients/
         clients about their right of access to their health
         records?   ☐   ☐
    iii Does the leaflet give a comprehensive account about
         who has got access to the patient's health record and
         how it is being used?   ☐   ☐
    iv   Has the leaflet been adjusted to account for the needs
         of minorities registered with your practice (for example,
         is it suitable for reading by disabled, ethnic minorities)? ☐   ☐

c   Are the practice mechanisms in place ensuring that members
    of staff respect patients' wishes appropriately and accurately
    when processing their personal data?   ☐   ☐

d   Are the practice mechanisms in place ensuring that patients
    have given informed consent prior to the processing of their
    personal data?   ☐   ☐

e   Has your PHCT performed patient surveys which investigate
    the effectiveness and patients' satisfaction with the
    communication strategy?   ☐   ☐

f   Is your PHCT able to deal with detailed patient questions
    on the processing of their data?   ☐   ☐

6 Staff contracts

a   Has every member of staff got a clause in their contract
    about their duty towards confidentiality and data security?   ☐   ☐

b Is the content of the clause about confidentiality and data
security in the staff contract appropriate by:
  i taking into account the member of staff's job role and
    responsibilities ☐ ☐
  ii mentioning security issues (e.g. non-sharing of
    passwords) ☐ ☐
  iii linking to disciplinary procedures in cases of breach of
    confidentiality? ☐ ☐

7 Contracts placed with other organisations
a Have you got a signed confidentiality undertaking agreement
with all contractors who carry out tasks in your practice? ☐ ☐
b Does the confidentiality undertaking agreement bind all
employees of the contractor and include any subcontractors? ☐ ☐
  i Does the contract allow the immediate termination in
    case of a breach of security or confidentiality? ☐ ☐
  ii Does the contract include that civil action might be taken
    and damage might be claimed against the contractor
    and/or his/her employee in case of a breach of security
    or confidentiality? ☐ ☐
c Have you got procedures/protocols in place that are aimed
to protect security and confidentiality beyond the contractor's
undertaking agreement, e.g.:
  i that everything feasible is done to remove confidential
    data from the contractor's working environment ☐ ☐
  ii that in case of work being undertaken posing a potential
    high risk to security or confidentiality accordingly
    stringent measures are put in place to minimise any
    chances of breaches of security and confidentiality? ☐ ☐

8 Reviewing information flows
a Has your practice mapped information flows/transfers of
information? ☐ ☐
Has the information flow/transfer been reviewed against the
Caldicott Principles, in particular:
  i does this information transfer serve a necessary purpose ☐ ☐
  ii is the minimum necessary patient-identifiable data in the
    information transfer? ☐ ☐
b Has the PHCT discussed the result of the review and if and
how changes could be made? ☐ ☐
c Is the review taking place on a regular (yearly) basis? ☐ ☐

9 Information/data 'ownership'
a Has each logical or physical set of confidential information
within your practice/PHCT been assigned to an 'owner'? ☐ ☐
  i Have all data sets (i.e. records, computers, letters) been
    identified within the practice? ☐ ☐
  ii Have you specified how the data set should only
    be used? ☐ ☐

b　Have you got an up-to-date register of all data 'owners'? □ □
　　i　Does the data owner understand his/her responsibilities
　　　towards his/her 'owned' data set? □ □
　　ii　Have those who should be authorised to have access to
　　　that data set been identified? □ □
c　Are all the data 'owners' working closely with their practice's
　　Caldicott Guardian? □ □
　　i　Are the purposes for holding those data justified? □ □
　　ii　Has the sensitivity of those data been determined and
　　　is access granted accordingly? □ □
　　iii　Is the data owner in proper control of who has access? □ □

10　Safe-haven procedures
　　a　Have you got written safe-haven policies and procedures
　　　for your practice? □ □
　　　i　Is every member of staff aware of the existence of these
　　　　safe-haven policies and procedures? □ □
　　　ii　Are these policies and procedures reviewed yearly? □ □
　　b　Have you got one designated and secured contact point in
　　　your practice through which confidential information is to be
　　　disclosed or accepted, i.e. coming in or leaving your practice? □ □
　　c　Do the safe-haven procedures cover all confidential
　　　information? □ □
　　d　Have you got a records management policy? □ □
　　　i　Does this policy contain guidance on data quality? □ □
　　　ii　Does this policy contain guidance on record retention? □ □

11　Protocols to govern information sharing
　　a　Have you identified all the organisations with which you
　　　disclose or exchange confidential patient-identifiable
　　　information (e.g. social services, police, education services
　　　and so on)? □ □
　　b　Are you following local PCT/PCO protocols on the
　　　disclosure or exchange of confidential information with
　　　these organisations? □ □
　　c　If there are no local PCT/PCO protocols, does the transfer
　　　of confidential information adhere to the following
　　　documented principles:
　　　i　that the use of the information is for an agreed and
　　　　legitimate purpose only □ □
　　　ii　that the disclosure is on a need-to-know basis □ □
　　　iii　that the receiving organisation is meeting the same
　　　　high standards on confidentiality and data security as
　　　　the NHS? □ □

12　Security policy
　　a　Does your practice have a written security policy? □ □
　　　i　Are all members of staff familiar with the security policy? □ □
　　　ii　Do all members of staff adhere to it? □ □
　　b　Is this security policy reviewed and updated yearly? □ □

    c   Is the security policy comprehensive and reach a minimum standard, i.e. does this policy include items such as:

       i   equipment security (including virus protection, backup procedures and physical security of equipment) ☐ ☐

      ii   equipment maintenance ☐ ☐

     iii   maintaining the confidentiality of all data within the practice ☐ ☐

     iv   disposal of confidential material and equipment ☐ ☐

      v   a protocol regarding the use and maintenance of CCTV equipment? ☐ ☐

13 Security responsibilities

    a   Has your PHCT an identified and clearly recognisable security lead on IM&T (may be the same person as the Caldicott Guardian)? ☐ ☐

    b   Has the IM&T security lead – if different person from the Caldicott Guardian – adequate training/knowledge in:

       i   the relevant legislation, e.g. Data Protection Act, and Caldicott requirements ☐ ☐

      ii   developing a comprehensive security policy ☐ ☐

     iii   leading on confidentiality and data security ☐ ☐

     iv   IM&T ☐ ☐

      v   safe-haven procedures ☐ ☐

     vi   data ownership? ☐ ☐

    c   Is the IM&T security lead – if different from the Caldicott Guardian – supported by all members of the PHCT? ☐ ☐

    d   Have you got a programme which raises awareness in matters of security and confidentiality? ☐ ☐

       i   Is a programme in place which raises awareness in matters of data and IM&T security and confidentiality? ☐ ☐

      ii   Are regular meetings within the PHCT taking place? ☐ ☐

     iii   Has a programme for audits been developed? ☐ ☐

14 Risk assessment and management

    a   Has your practice performed a risk assessment and developed a risk management strategy? ☐ ☐

    b   Are the undertaken risk assessment and the developed risk management strategy comprehensive and documented? ☐ ☐

       i   Has a full inventory been completed? ☐ ☐

      ii   Has each item of the inventory been assessed for the possibility of a security threat? ☐ ☐

     iii   Has each item of the inventory been assessed for the impact it would have in the case of an adverse event? ☐ ☐

     iv   Has the vulnerability been determined in the case of an adverse event? ☐ ☐

    c   Have you developed an action plan following the outcome of the risk assessment? ☐ ☐

       i   Have you agreed on this action plan among all the main stakeholders in the PHCT? ☐ ☐

ii   Have you established a programme for regular risk
assessment within the action plan?   □   □

15   Security incidents
a   Has your PHCT established a reporting system for
security incidents?   □   □
    i   Does every member of staff know what is meant by a
    'security incident'?   □   □
    ii   Does every member of staff know to whom to report a
    security incident?   □   □
    iii Have you got a security incident report pro-forma? □   □
    iv   Have all the security incidents been documented and
    logged/filed?   □   □
b   Have you got written guidance on how to deal with a
security incident?   □   □
    i   Is the guidance known and understood by every member
    of staff?   □   □
    ii   Is the guidance easily accessible for any member of staff? □   □
c   Are procedures in place that aim to improve security after a
security incident?   □   □
    i   Are security incidents discussed at team meetings? □   □
    ii   Are policies and guidelines investigated and possibly
    amended and then distributed to every member of staff
    following a security incident?   □   □

16   Security monitoring
a   Does your PHCT review the effectiveness of security
measures?   □   □
    i   Are all members of staff involved in meetings that
    monitor security?   □   □
    ii   Are all aspects of security monitored: potential and
    actual security breaches, compliance with existing
    guidelines, e.g. log-on and log-off procedures, use of
    passwords, safe-haven procedures and so on?   □   □
    iii Are reports on security discussed during these meetings
    and outcomes documented?   □   □
    iv   Are outcomes of these meetings well distributed to
    every member of staff?   □   □
b   Are you monitoring the effectiveness of your security
measures on a regular (yearly) basis?   □   □

17   User responsibilities
a   Does your PHCT have a written policy on the
responsibilities of users of IM&T equipment?   □   □
b   Does this policy cover:
    i   the use of passwords, when to change and how to
    construct them   □   □
    ii   clear desk, clear screen policy   □   □
    iii how to deal with and report potential or actual security
    breaches   □   □

      iv issues regarding the maintenance of IM&T equipment
          such as virus protection, data input, use of stored data?   ☐ ☐

  c Does every member of staff that uses IM&T equipment
     understand the written policies about his/her responsibilities? ☐ ☐

  d Are checks performed on a regular (yearly) basis to see if these
     responsibilities are adhered to?   ☐ ☐

18 Access controls
  a Is the physical access to confidential data and material
     controlled?   ☐ ☐
  b Is the logical access to confidential data controlled?   ☐ ☐
     i Are steps undertaken to prevent data misuse?   ☐ ☐
     ii Are users of computers registered and de-registered as
        their position within the team changes?   ☐ ☐
     iii Have you got written guidance on passwords?   ☐ ☐
     iv Have you got a good standard for log-on and log-off
        procedures?   ☐ ☐
  c Has your PHCT got a written policy on third-party access
     to confidential data/material?   ☐ ☐

Having performed your information governance assessment every item of the questionnaire that is not ticked as YES should be considered as an area in need of improvement.

When developing an action plan it will be important to be aware of a realistic timeframe to achieve your goals and the financial implications of the proposed action plan for the following year (*see* also Section 20, Implementation strategy).

Audits should be performed yearly to monitor progress, ensure the maintaining of the standard once reached and overall to improve data protection, security and confidentiality.

Reference

1 IG Toolkit: http://www.nhsia.nhs.uk/infogov/igt/RequirementsList.

Section 20
Implementation strategy

This section aims to help in developing a strategy on how to improve on your information governance by introducing the Caldicott requirements[1] and standards of the Data Protection Act[2] into the working lives of your PHCT and to help in formalising this process as well as documenting that all the standards have been achieved. Your strategy may also incorporate issues discussed in Chapters 2 and 3.

Starting from the beginning to introduce information governance in your PHCT

The following steps are suggestions on the basis that, for only a little amount of time and effort spent, quick gains can be achieved. The further down the list you get, the more effort will need to be invested to achieve the Caldicott requirements.

1   Nominate a Caldicott Guardian/information governance lead in your PHCT (for simplicity the following text will only refer to this person as Caldicott Guardian). It should be a senior health professional or be closely supported by such a person (e.g. GP or practice manager).[3,4] The remit of the role of such a person is outlined in Section 1, Caldicott Guardian/Information Governance Lead.
2   Check if all the staff contracts have got a signed confidentiality undertaking (an example of the wording of such a confidentiality undertaking can be found in Section 6, Staff contracts). Print the relevant wording from www.radcliffe-oxford.com/informationgov, or reword it according to your needs and, after it has been signed by the member of staff, attach it to the existing contract.
3   Give every 'new patient' the patient information leaflet 'Protecting and using your personal and medical information' and use the poster to publicise patients' rights (*see* Section 5, Communication with patients/information for patients). Print the wording from www.radcliffe-oxford.com/informationgov, or reword it according to your needs/circumstances.
4   Every member of staff should receive a copy of the following documents (therefore print the wording from www.radcliffe-oxford.com/informationgov, or reword it according to your needs or circumstances):
     a   staff code of conduct in respect of patient confidentiality (*see* Section 2)
     b   safe-haven procedures (Section 10)
     c   security policy (Section 12)
     d   user responsibilities (Section 17)
     e   access controls (Section 18).

5   Assess and document on a yearly basis the confidentiality and security training needs of every member of staff (*see* Section 4).
6   Nominate 'data owners' for every logical data unit according to the guidelines about information/data 'ownership' (*see* Section 9). Print from www.radcliffe-oxford.com/informationgov the suggested form of register, adjust it to your practice and collect the signatures of the 'data owners' before filing it for future reference.

7　The practice's Caldicott Guardian should be aware of the security respon-sibilities and establish safe-haven procedures including the records manage-ment policy (*see* Sections 13 and 10).

8　The practice's Caldicott Guardian should encourage the reporting of security incidents and monitor the effectiveness of and compliance with security poli-cies (*see* Sections 15 and 16).

9　The practice's Caldicott Guardian needs to undertake a risk assessment and develop the resulting risk management plan (*see* Section 14, Risk assessment and management).

10　The reviewing of information flows (*see* Section 8) is a time-consuming but important task as it aims to ensure/improve the patient's privacy when data are transferred.

11　Non-NHS organisations contracted to perform tasks within the premises or for the PHCT should sign a confidentiality undertaking (*see* Section 7, Contracts placed with other organisations). You might like to print these confidentiality agreements from www.radcliffe-oxford.com/informationgov.

12　The practice's Caldicott Guardian is responsible for the proper introduc-tion of new members of staff. This means not only that the staff induction procedures need to be formalised but also that a training needs assessment should be undertaken, as well as their access to confidential information determined (*see* Sections 3, 4 and 18). You might like to print the checklist and form for registration from www.radcliffe-oxford.com/informationgov.

Having established information governance in your PHCT

When developing an action plan it will be important to be aware of a realistic time-frame to achieve your goals and the financial implications of the proposed action plan for the coming year (*see* also Section 19, Information governance assessment).

Audits should be performed yearly to monitor progress, ensure the maintaining of the standard once reached and overall to improve data protection, security and confidentiality.

Things to do on regular (annual) basis:

* notification to the Information Commissioner up to date
* perform an information governance audit
* review practice leaflet
* review of data flow
* risk assessment
* update policies
* training
* patient satisfaction surveys.

When you propose changes check:

* if it will be realistic to achieve
* the financial impact of the change so it will be 'value for money'
* the training needs to introduce the changes

- the time commitment and motivation of members of staff
- which measures are needed to take to evaluate if the changes achieved their proposed effect.

References

1 DoH (1999) *Protecting and Using Patient Information: a manual for Caldicott Guardians*, March.
2 *See* Chapter 2.
3 DoH (1997) *The Caldicott Committee Report on the Review of Patient-identifiable Information*, December, Recommendation 3. http://www.hmso.gov.uk/confiden/app2.htm
4 HSC 1999/012: *Caldicott Guardians*.

Chapter 2

Data Protection Act 1998

The Data Protection Principles[1]

The Data Protection Principles (which are derived from the Data Protection Act 1998) increase the responsibility of anyone who processes personal data, strengthen the individual's right to privacy, and ensure that the processing of personal data is done in accordance with the rights of individuals.
    The Principles state the following:

1   The information to be contained in personal data shall be obtained, and personal data shall be processed, fairly and lawfully and shall not be processed unless certain conditions apply.
2   Personal data shall be held only for one or more specified and lawful purposes.
3   Personal data held for any purpose or purposes shall be adequate, relevant and not excessive in relation to that purpose or those purposes.
4   Personal data shall be accurate and, where necessary, kept up to date.
5   Personal data held for any purpose or purposes shall not be kept for longer than is necessary for that purpose or purposes.
6   Personal data shall be processed in accordance with the rights of the data subject under this Act, e.g. an individual shall be entitled

   a   to be informed by any data user whether he holds personal data of which that individual is the subject and
   b   to have access to any such data held by a data user, at reasonable intervals and without undue delay or expense
   c   to have such data corrected or erased where appropriate.

7   Appropriate security measures shall be taken against unauthorised access to, or alteration, disclosure or destruction of personal data and against accidental loss or destruction of personal data.
8   Personal data shall not be transferred to a country or territory outside the European Economic Area unless there are adequate levels of protection for the rights of a data subject.

Explanatory notes about the Data Protection Principles

The following explanatory notes to the Data Protection Act 1998 (DPA) are not intended to be comprehensive but rather are selected according to their relevance to the PHCT. They give a summary of the official commentary. If there is any need for further clarification please refer to the Information Commissioner's Office website: http://www.informationcommissioner.gov.uk.

The First Principle

Personal data shall be processed fairly and lawfully and, in particular, shall not be processed unless:

- *at least one of the conditions in Schedule 2 is met, and*
- *in the case of sensitive personal data at least one of the conditions in Schedule 3 is also met.*

'Processing' under the new Act is defined as any activity undertaken with the information or data such as obtaining, recording or holding, or carrying out any operation or set of operations. It is a very broad definition and therefore includes virtually every type of activity involving data.

'Fairly and lawfully' means that

1 the data controller (who is (are) the person(s) deciding on the purpose(s) for which and the manner in which the data are processed e.g. doctor, nurse, health visitor or counsellor) has to comply with the common law duty of confidentiality and has a legitimate reason to process personal data; in the vast majority of cases this includes the patient's informed consent[2]
2 the data subject (who is the living individual e.g. the patient, relative or carer to whom the data is related) understands and agrees who will process the data, how they will be processed and for what purpose(s)
3 the data were obtained in a way that was neither misleading nor deceiving
4 unless justified for example by a legal/statutory requirement or significant public interest, the processing of patient (data subject) information is only justified by informed consent.[3]

'Schedule 2 and 3' define the conditions of processing data.[1] Personal data/health data may only be processed if at least one condition of Schedule 2 *and* one of Schedule 3 has been met. In addition the data controller must comply with other relevant laws as well.

Schedule 2 defines that *personal data* may be processed if

- the data subject has given his/her consent or
- the processing is necessary because

  − it is in the vital interest of the data subject
  − of a legal obligation

– of a statutory obligation
– of a legitimate interest of the data controller
– it is in the public interest
– a contract.

Schedule 3 specifies conditions of processing *sensitive* data if

- the data subject has given his/her explicit consent or
- the processing is necessary because

  – of medical purposes by health professionals
  – it is in the vital interests of the data subject where consent cannot be obtained
  – it is in the vital interest of another person where a consent cannot be obtained
  – of, or in connection with, legal proceedings
  – it serves the prevention or detection of an unlawful act
  – of substantial public interest
  – of legal obligations related to employment purposes or

- the data is processed in circumstances specified in an order issued by the Secretary of State or
- the processing is carried out in the course of legitimate activities of certain non-profit making organisations.

According to the view of the Data Protection Registrar/Commissioner the normal basis of processing of any health/sensitive data may be the implied consent but in certain circumstances should be the explicit/expressed consent.

The DPA allows the processing of personal data if consent has been given but the DPA does not define the term consent. Besides the European Union (EU) Directive's definition of consent,[4] the Information Commissioner set up guidance for what would constitute a valid consent.[5] According to the Information Commissioner the consent from the data subject must

- be informed. He or she must be given 'fair processing information'. This means the data subject must understand

  – who is the data controller
  – the proposed use(s) of his or her personal data
  – who else will get to know, i.e. to whom the personal data will be disclosed
  – any other necessary information which is specifically relevant to the processing of his or her personal data.

  This implies that the data subject must understand

  – what data is recorded and why
  – the benefit of the disclosure of personal data and the future uses of the data besides the risks, outcomes and implications if consent is withheld
  – how long it will be held and under which circumstances the information is destroyed
  – that any consent can be withdrawn in the future (however, it might be difficult to withdraw information which already has been shared).

- have some degree of choice. This means that under certain circumstances it is possible to attach a condition to the consent. In other words a valid consent does not necessarily have to be unconditional. For example, under certain circumstances the GP might ask the patient to consent to the disclosure of personal data to the PCO in return for the treatment which requires special financial support by the PCO.
- be given by some degree of indication. The lack of any response to any form of communication cannot be taken or seen as the data subject's given consent. To some degree an active communication should take place either by explicit or implied consent. Generally an implied consent is as valid as an expressed/ explicit consent.[6] It very much depends on the circumstances as to which type of consent should be preferred. Given that the expressed consent is less likely to be ambiguous or be misunderstood its use is required when for example the use(s) of information has changed from the time of collection and therefore 'fair processing information' was not given at that time.

Respecting the requirements of a valid consent it is clear that the blanket consent to processing of personal data would most likely be insufficient. It depends on the nature of the processing whether the consent should cover the details and the purpose of the processing as well as the type of data which are to be processed and how this may affect the data subject. Not only should the patient be informed about the consequences of the processing of his or her personal data but also the patient's wishes should be reflected.

Furthermore a consent is only valid if it is not based on misleading information. Once given, the consent will not necessarily be valid forever.

The PHCT should provide patients with leaflets that explain how their personal data are handled by the PHCT (*see* Chapter 1, Section 5, Communication with patients/information for patients). This should lead to a greater transparency on why and how personal data are used, stored and disclosed; however, fair processing information might have to be given besides distributing leaflets and putting up posters on confidentiality.

The Second Principle

Personal data shall be obtained only for one or more specified and lawful purposes, and shall not be further processed in any manner incompatible with that purpose or those purposes.

This principle intends to make the processing of personal data more transparent for the data subject and restricts the data controller's processing of personal data by limiting it to the specified purpose(s).

The disclosure of personal data by the data controller has to be compatible with the purpose for which the data subject has disclosed them originally. In other words, the confidential information obtained for one purpose cannot be used for any other purposes, unless consent is sought or exemptions apply, for example if there is an overriding public interest or a requirement of the law.

In general the data controller is still obliged to give 'fair processing information' even though the disclosure of personal data is justified without consent of the data subject. The exemptions to this rule are only situations in which it would be inconsistent with the disclosure to give the patient fair processing information.

Examples
- Fair processing information should be given although disclosure does not require the consent of the patient. For example, a GP reports a patient's diagnosed cancer to a cancer register under section 60 of the Health and Social Care Act.[7] The GP continues to have the duty to inform the patient of the disclosure of his/her personal data and its consequences even though the clinician did not require the patient's consent for this disclosure.
- Section 29 of the DPA permits the disclosure of personal data for the purpose of the prevention or detection of crime or the prosecution of offenders and is an example of circumstances in which the requirement to give fair processing information does not apply because giving the data subject fair processing information might prejudice the purpose of the disclosure.

Furthermore the data controller should ensure that those to whom the confidential information is disclosed will not use it for any other purpose(s) than for the original disclosure.

The Third Principle

Personal data shall be adequate, relevant and not excessive in relation to the purpose or purposes for which they are processed.

Personal data should not be collected from a data subject which are not relevant at the time they were collected but might be 'handy' in the future. There is a great risk in such cases that fair processing information is not given appropriately as the use(s) of those personal data were not determined at the time they were collected.

The Fourth Principle

Personal data shall be accurate and, where necessary, kept up to date.
Data are inaccurate if they are incorrect or misleading as to any matter of fact.

According to the guidance in interpreting this principle it may no longer be sufficient for a data controller to claim that the data were obtained from the data subject as the data controller may have to go further and take reasonable steps to ensure that the data themselves are accurate.

The data controller has to ensure as well that personal data from the data subject are recorded accurately. There are multiple means to ensure the accuracy of the data: for example, while entering information into the patient's records double-check with the patient its accuracy or let the patient read his/her own records while waiting for a consultation.

A policy on data quality as part of the records management policy is outlined in Chapter 1, Section 10, Safe-haven procedures.

Furthermore, if the data subject expresses the view that any data held by the data controller are incorrect then the data controller should indicate that fact in those data.

The Fifth Principle

Personal data processed for any purpose(s) shall not be kept for longer than is necessary for that purpose or those purpose(s).

The PHCT will need to review its compliance with legal requirements on retention periods of records and will need to develop protocols on the retention and disposal of records. *See* the policy on records management in Chapter 1, Section 10, Safe-haven procedures.

The Sixth Principle

Personal data shall be processed in accordance with the rights of data subjects under this Act.

Here again the Act gives guidance in interpreting this principle. A data controller will contravene this principle if the data controller fails to

- comply with the individual's rights (*see* Chapter 1, Section 2, Staff code of conduct)
- supply information following a subject's access request
- comply with a notice to rectify, block, erase or destroy inaccurate data
- prevent the processing of data notified as likely to cause damage or distress
- prevent direct marketing of data
- comply with a notice in relation to automated decision making.

The automated decision making might be of particular relevance to the PHCT. The PHCT must review its IM&T system to find out whether or not the software utilises automated decision making. If the IT system utilises automated decision making the PHCT needs to ensure that it complies with the data protection requirements and if necessary make appropriate changes.

The patient has to be notified by the data controller if a decision is based solely on automatic processing and can have a serious effect on that individual.

The Seventh Principle

Appropriate technical and organisational measures shall be taken against unauthorised or unlawful processing of personal data and against acci-dental loss or destruction of, or damage to personal data.

This principle puts the obligation upon the data controllers to introduce a whole host of measures. These measures should mirror the potential harm which could result from a breach of security and since a PHCT collects highly sensitive data there is a great need to put adequate procedures in place. The PHCT should

- have a security policy (*see* Chapter 1, Section 12)
- have risk assessment and management procedures (*see* Chapter 1, Section 14)
- have protocols regarding security incidents (*see* Chapter 1, Section 15)
- have security monitoring procedures (*see* Chapter 1, Section 16)
- have safe-haven procedures (*see* Chapter 1, Section 10)
- ensure staff access is controlled (*see* Chapter 1, Section 18) and staff reliability which means

  - following guidelines on IT security (*see* Chapter 1, Sections 13 and 17)
  - complying with the code of conduct in respect to confidentiality (*see* Chapter 1, Section 2)
  - having staff induction procedures (*see* Chapter 1, Section 3) and reviewing training needs (*see* Chapter 1, Section 4)
  - having confidentiality agreements in staff contracts (*see* Chapter 1, Section 6)
  - complying with Caldicott Principles.[8]

The Eighth Principle

Personal data shall not be transferred to a country or territory outside the European Economic Area, unless that country or territory ensures an adequate level for the rights and freedoms of data subjects in relation to the processing of personal data.

If a matter arises that falls under the regulation of this principle, further assistance, e.g. from the Medical Defence Union/Medical Protection Society, would most likely be required.

Individuals' rights

The Data Protection Act 1998 gives data subjects (i.e. patients, clients, carers) certain rights in respect to their own personal data held in any form (computer and/or paper records)[1]

- the right of access to their personal data
- the right to prevent the processing of data likely to cause damage or distress
- rights when automated decision making is used by the data controller (e.g. the data subject must be informed about the logic involved in the automated decision making)
- the right to take action for compensation if the individual suffers damage
- the right to take action (i.e. rectify, block, erase or destroy data) in cases where inaccurate data exist.

The right of access to personal data

Right of application

The right of application is owned

- by any living patient in writing (records of deceased persons are still governed by the Access to the Health Records Act 1990); proof of identification can be requested
- by a competent child (Fraser Guidelines apply)[9]
- by a child's natural parents or applicant who has got parental responsibility
- by any person, authorised in writing, to apply on behalf of the patient
- by any person, appointed by the court, to manage affairs of a patient
- by a solicitor or the police having gained a court order.

No reason and no time specification need to be given.

Personal data

- Personal data include any health records (i.e. not only handwritten or computerised clinical notes but also letters to and from health professionals, x-rays and their reports, videos, tape recordings, conversations, computer printouts, laboratory results, 'private'/non-NHS records etc.).
- There is no time limit, i.e. it does not matter when the data were compiled.
- Access should be given to all the data contained at the time when the request was received.
- Routine amendments and deletions of data may continue between the date of request and the reply; however, no deletion or special amendments should be made which would otherwise not have been made.

Dealing with the access request

- Under the Data Protection Act 1998 the obligation to provide access rests with the holder of the record, i.e. the data controller who is the GP.

- After receiving a written (or in any other permanent form) application the request should be dealt with within 40 days.
- A fee may be charged.
- There should be a reasonable interval between requests.
- Where the information is not readily intelligible an explanation must be given (for example, abbreviations or medical terminology).

When the access to records may be denied or partially excluded

- If the information could be damaging to the patient himself/herself (physically or mentally) or any other person it can be withheld; the record holder does not have to volunteer the fact that the records are incomplete because of the above reason.
- Where the applicant is not the patient and the holder of the record is of the opinion that the patient gave the information/investigation/examination in the expectation that the information would not be disclosed to the applicant.
- If the applicant is not capable of understanding the nature of the application or the meaning of the authorisation.
- If there has not been a reasonable interval since previous compliance with an access request.
- The fee has not been paid.
- If access to data may result in disclosing information relating to or provided by a third party (this does not include any healthcare professionals) who had not consented to the disclosure but can be identified from that information. In such cases criteria must be:

  – the third party gives his/her consent or
  – it is reasonable in all circumstances to comply with the request without the consent of the third party when

    ○ steps are taken to obtain their consent
    ○ the third party is capable of giving consent

  – the data controller must, however, give as much information as possible without identifying the third party if consent is deemed to be necessary but cannot be obtained.

The denial of access is not justified because of

- fear of litigation or any other legal action
- the cost of giving access being higher than the maximum chargeable fee.

Access to health records of deceased persons

- This is regulated by the Access to Health Records Act 1990.
- When the patient has died, his/her personal representative or executor or administrator or anyone having a claim resulting from the death has the right to apply for access to the deceased's records.

- The request should be made in writing.
- If the deceased person had indicated that he/she did not wish information to be disclosed, or the record contains information that the deceased person expected to remain confidential, then it cannot be disclosed.
- The record holder has the right to deny or restrict the access if he/she feels that the disclosure would cause serious physical or mental harm to any other person or would identify a third person. This does not include healthcare professionals.

You might like to print this protocol from www.radcliffe-oxford.com/information gov on your practice's letter headed paper.

Protocol for access to health records

Patient's name: _____

Address: _____

DoB: _____ / _____ / _____

Date of application: _____ / _____ / _____

Is the applicant the patient: Yes/No

If NO, what are the legal reasons for this request: _____

_____

_____

Reasons for access being denied or partially excluded:

Yes/No

If YES, please record reason: _____

_____

_____

Date of releasing copy: _____ / _____ / _____

Applicant's identity confirmed by means of: _____

_____

Signature: _____ Date: _____ / _____ / _____

(Practice's Caldicott Guardian/practice manager/GP)

The right to take action in cases where inaccurate data exist

- If the patient claims that there are mistakes/inaccuracies in the records or if the patient feels that they are misleading to any matter of fact(s), the patient can ask the record holder to make a note stating this opinion.
- The note should be made at the relevant place.
- If the record holder agrees that there is a true mistake regarding any matter of fact, then the mistake should be corrected and
- the data controller should make reasonable efforts to notify third parties to whom the data have been disclosed of the rectification, blocking, erasure or destruction of any data.
- If the data are incorrect but accurately record the information given to the data controller by the data subject or a third party; the data controller still has to prove that he respected his duty set out in the Fourth Principle (the data controller has to take reasonable steps to ensure that the data are correct – independent of their source).

CCTV and Commissioner's Code of Practice (section 51(3)(b) DPA 1998)[1]

The Data Protection Act provides the grounds for legally enforceable standards that apply to the collection and processing of images of individuals. This means that the use of closed circuit television (CCTV) is now clearly regulated, giving the operators of CCTV clear guidance and understanding of their legal obligations.[10]

The following describes the standards and gives the protocols which would be most likely applicable to a practice operating CCTV.

The standards applicable are the same as for any other collected data and are spelt out at the beginning of Chapter 2, the Data Protection Principles. According to these principles the following has to be observed.

1   Before establishing a CCTV scheme the appropriateness of it, the reasons for it, and the purpose for its use must be documented, e.g.:

 a   its use for the prevention and detection of crime within the premises of the practice
 b   its use for the safety of patients/carers, visitors and staff of the practice.

 The CCTV equipment should only be used to achieve the purposes set out above. Therefore the cameras should be positioned in order to achieve these purposes. Neighbouring property may only be covered after consultations with its owner.

2   The organisation and/or person(s) who are legally responsible for the CCTV scheme, and, if different to those legally responsible, also the organisation/person(s) who is (are) responsible for the daily running of the scheme has (have) to be nominated and documented.

3   A notification should be lodged with the office of the Data Protection Commissioner which must provide the information above.

4   Accompanying the CCTV scheme should be a documented security policy (*see* also Chapter 1, Section 12; Security policy), and a designated senior member of staff (e.g. Caldicott Guardian, practice manager, GP) should be put in charge of the security policy.

5   Signs must be positioned in areas covered by the surveillance equipment. These signs must be clearly visible and easy to read for the public, appropriate in size and contain the following information:

 a   warning that the area is covered by CCTV
 b   the purpose of the surveillance
 c   who or which organisation is responsible for that scheme
 d   whom to contact for further information.

 A sign could have the following wording:

> This area is covered by CCTV for crime prevention and the safety of visitors and staff of this surgery. This scheme is controlled by Busy Doctors Surgery. For information contact Tel 0222 2222.

6   Images should not be retained for longer than is necessary.

7   The practice is obliged to have a policy on the disclosure of images. Access to the images should be strictly controlled and documented. It should be a

designated senior member of the practice staff who is in charge of controlling the access to CCTV images and finding the location of the images.

8   If access has been denied, the person who requested the access should be given the reasons why the request has been denied in writing and the practice's complaints procedures.

The following are proposed policies on security and disclosure that might need to be altered and extended to cover the needs of your practice. Finally this section provides application and reply forms which could be used in the case of a request to have access to CCTV images – again you might like to alter these forms to adapt them to suit your needs.

You might want to print the following from www.radcliffe-oxford.com/informationgov on your practice's letter-headed paper:

Security policy for CCTV surveillance

(Name) _____ is the designated member of staff who is in charge of and responsible for the following security policy for CCTV and the regular monitoring of its effectiveness.

In the absence of the above-named person (Name) _____ is in charge of the security policy.

The security policy aims to ensure that the obligations and responsibilities set out in the Commissioner's Code of Practice (section 51(3)(b) of the Data Protection Act 1998) are achieved.

The CCTV equipment is regularly reviewed by the above-named person to guarantee it achieves its purpose for crime protection and public safety, i.e. camera(s) are located to observe only the area intended for surveillance, to be protected from vandalism and physical interference, that it functions properly, that tapes are of good quality and replaced on a regular basis and that images are clear (and if applicable with reference to location of camera and date and time).

The above-named person ensures the maintenance of the equipment, that it is serviced according to specification: ensuring the upkeep, cleaning, timely repair and replacement of faulty equipment and documentation by an up-to-date log-book.

The above-named person ensures the safety of recorded images, that they are locked up and not kept longer than necessary and that as soon as the images are not required any more (normally about seven days unless special circumstances apply) they are removed or erased.

The above-named person has the responsibility of ensuring that access to the images is strictly controlled only to authorised members of staff and any access documented and in line with the disclosure policy, and that the monitor(s) is (are) positioned so it (they) can be overlooked only by designated staff.

Disclosure policy for recorded CCTV images

(Name) _____ is the designated member of staff who is in charge of and responsible for the following disclosure policy for CCTV images and the regular monitoring of its effectiveness.

In the absence of the above-named person (Name) _____ is in charge of the disclosure policy.

The disclosure policy aims to ensure that the obligations and responsibilities set out in the Commissioner's Code of Practice (section 51(3)(b) of the Data Protection Act 1998) are met.

Access to recorded images/CCTV should be restricted to those members of staff who need to have access to achieve its defined purpose.

The above-named person is responsible for documenting all requests to access to stored images and any actual access to stored images should be documented.

The above-named person will ensure that disclosure of recorded images to a third party is limited to special circumstances according to the code of practice for CCTV and that, prior to disclosure of CCTV images, any third party whose image is not to be disclosed will have his/her image disguised or blurred.

Any applicants who request access to CCTV images will be provided with the code of practice, application form for access, and in case access has been denied the practice's leaflet on complaints procedures.

Code of practice for CCTV

_____
Name of practice

The purpose of the CCTV surveillance is for the prevention and detection of crime within the premises of the practice and for the safety of patients/carers, visitors and staff of the practice.

_____ is legally responsible for
Name of practice or person responsible for scheme
the CCTV scheme.

_____ is responsible for the day-
Name of practice or person responsible for scheme
to-day running of the CCTV surveillance scheme.

_____ has notified the Office of
Name of practice or person
the Data Protection Commissioner about the operation of the CCTV surveillance scheme.

The cameras are positioned to achieve solely the purpose of the surveillance scheme and therefore only cover the following areas:

_____.

_____.

Signs are placed in the zone covered by the surveillance informing the public about the use of CCTV and are positioned to be clearly visible and legible in the following areas:

_____.

_____.

_____ is in charge of the security policy for
Name (practice Caldicott Guardian/GP/practice manager)
CCTV, oversees its implementation and monitors compliance.

Application by a third party for the disclosure of CCTV images

The Data Protection Act 1998 demands that the disclosure of recorded images to a third party should be limited to the purpose for which they were originally obtained. The CCTV surveillance operated by this practice is for the prevention and detection of crime within the premises of the practice and for the safety of patients, carers, visitors and staff of the practice and images may be released only to achieve these purposes.

Please state the reason for your request to have access to the recorded images:

_____

_____

_____

_____ .

Date and time when images where taken: /   /___   ____ :___
(for location purposes)

Name of person requesting access: _____ .

Job title: _____

Date of request: /   /___

Address/police station: _____

_____

_____

Signature of applicant: _____

Practice's reply to the request for the disclosure of CCTV images by a third party

Reason(s) to grant/not to grant the request:

_____

_____

_____

Extent to which disclosure was allowed:

_____

_____

_____

Crime incident number: _____

Location of images: _____

Identity of applicant verified by means: _____

Date when images were removed: ___ / ___ / _____

Signature: (of collecting applicant if applicable) _____

Images of individuals not related to the investigation/incident have been disguised prior to the release of the tape.

Signature: _____
         (Practice Caldicott Guardian/practice manager/GP)

Application by a data subject for the disclosure of CCTV images

The CCTV surveillance operated by this practice is for the prevention and detection of crime within the premises of the practice and for the safety of patients, carers, visitors and staff of the practice and images may be released only to achieve these purposes. Images are normally destroyed after seven days.

Please state the reason for your request to have access to the recorded images:

_____

_____

_____

_____.

Date and time when images where taken: ___ / ___ / ___   ___ : ___
(for location purposes)

Means of identification of person making request: _____

Name and address of person requesting access: _____

_____

_____

_____.

Date of request: ___ / ___ / ___

Request to view/have a copy of the images.
(please circle as appropriate)

I am aware that a fee of max. £10 may be charged to carry out the search to locate the images. Once the fee has been received it will take a maximum of 40 days for a response.

Signature of applicant: _____

Practice's reply to the request for the disclosure of CCTV images by a data subject

Reason(s) to grant/not to grant the request:

_____

_____

_____

Extent to which disclosure was allowed:

_____

_____

_____

Location of images: _____

Identity of applicant verified by means: _____

Date when images were removed: ___/___/___

Images of individuals not related to the investigation/incident have been disguised prior to the release of the tape.

Signature: _____
(Practice Caldicott Guardian/practice manager/GP)

References

1   Data Protection Act 1998: http://www.hmso.gov.uk/acts/acts1998/1998 0029.htm and http://www.informationcommissioner.gov.uk.

2   The GMC provides detailed guidance on consent on its website: http://www/gmc-uk.org/standards/.

3   For advice on exceptional circumstances when the requirement for informed consent may be overridden *see* also BMA Ethical Committee (1999) *Confidentiality and Disclosure of Health Information*, October.

4   EU Directive 95/46/EC.

5   Information Commissioner (2002) *Use and Disclosure of Health Data: guidance on the application of the Data Protection Act 1998*, May. http://www.informationcommissioner.gov.uk

6   GMC (2004) *Confidentiality: protecting and providing information.* http://www.gmc-uk.org/standards/

7   Only applicable in England and Wales.

8   DoH (1997) *The Caldicott Committee Report on the Review of Patient-identifiable Information*, December. http://www.hmso.gov.uk/confiden/app2.htm

9   The judgement offered in Gillick vs West Norfolk and Wisbech AHA & DHSS in 1985 is now referred to as the Fraser Guidelines.

10   http://www.informationcommissioner.gov.uk

Chapter 3

Other important legislation and guidance

Common law duty of confidentiality[1]

The common law duty of confidentiality was built up from case law based on individual judgements. It is not regulated by any Act of Parliament. Everyone is subject to the common law duty of confidentiality and must abide by it. It relates to all person-identifiable information which is not in the public domain, which is of a certain degree of sensitivity and has been provided in confidence for a particular purpose. The common law duty of confidentiality does not relate to effectively anonymised information, i.e. any information that is not possible for anyone to link to a specific individual.

The common law duty of confidentiality does not always provide a concept that is easy to follow and to apply because

- certain areas have not been litigated and therefore it remains unclear if a duty of confidentiality exists
- as the NHS modernises and changes, some of the decisions made by courts in the past might not apply today
- there are not always general concepts and rules which can be derived from previous cases.

The key principle of the common law duty of confidentiality is that information received should not be used or disclosed in any other way than originally understood and consented to by the confider, or unless subsequent permission is received. Disclosure or use of personal data without consent may only be permitted in exceptional circumstances, such as a significant public interest or a legal/statutory requirement.[2]

The law is not very clear as to whether the common law duty of confidentiality also extends to the deceased. However, the DoH and professional bodies[3] are of the opinion that a deceased person is also protected by the common law duty of confidentiality.

Human Rights Act 1998[4]

The Human Rights Act (HRA) 1998, which came into force in the United Kingdom in 2000, incorporates the Protection of Human Rights and Fundamental Freedoms set out in the European Convention on Human Rights. Although the current understanding is that through compliance with the Data Protection Act

1998 and especially with the common law duty of confidentiality the HRA requirements are satisfied, the full effect of the HRA has yet to be established by the English courts, which will also need to take into account decisions of the European Court of Human Rights.

The HRA applies to public authorities, which have a duty to ensure that their actions do not contravene the HRA by either interfering with the rights of the individual or by failing to protect these rights. Under the HRA an individual can only take a public authority to court, not another individual or body. However, there is a significant indirect effect if a protected human right is contravened by another individual or body because the court might find that existing legislation did not sufficiently protect the rights of the individual. Since a general practice is not a public authority it can not be taken to court for not complying with the HRA.

The most important Articles of the HRA which might apply to the conduct of NHS staff/employees towards patients are Articles 8 and 14:

> Article 8: The right to respect for private and family life
>
> This Article underpins the Data Protection Act 1998. Unauthorised disclosure of patient-identifiable information would constitute a breach of this Article, unless legitimate exemptions apply such as e.g. the protection of public safety, the prevention of crime and disorder etc.
>
> Article 14: The prohibition of discrimination
>
> This Article emphasises the duty of the NHS to embrace all patients, which includes any minority. It would be a contravention of the HRA if e.g. information about the use and access to health records is provided in a way so that minorities (i.e. patients who cannot speak English, have learning disabilities, are blind) are not able to understand it.

Crime and Disorder Act 1998

The Crime and Disorder Act introduces several measures which require the police and local authorities to work together with other agencies to develop and implement a strategy that reduces crime and disorder through the introduction of local crime partnerships for the delivery of safer communities.

This has a knock-on effect on the way patient-identifiable information is handled as the Act facilitates the exchange of information between agencies as they are given responsibilities for the wider community. Although the Crime and Disorder Act does not in itself constitute a statutory requirement for a general practice/PHCT to disclose patient information, it is important that a general practice/PHCT is in full support of and contributes to the local crime partnerships while respecting the constraints provided by common and statutory law. In other words the Act allows the disclosure of patient-identifiable information by the PHCT (for the purposes of the Act) to other organisations such as the police, local authorities, probation services, but the responsibility for the disclosure will rest with the PHCT holding the information.[5] The PHCT will always need to operate within legal requirements and restraints such as the Data Protection Act and the common law duty of confidentiality. However, there are no such restrictions on effectively anonymised data as the common law duty of confidentiality does not apply to such information.

There are significant numbers of opportunities in which a PHCT might play a key role in reducing crime such as domestic violence, child abuse etc. It is therefore paramount that PHCTs and PCOs develop crime and disorder protocols that regulate and provide guidance on information sharing.

The crime and disorder protocols for information sharing

- should spell out the legal requirements to be observed when sharing information
- should define the purpose for sharing the information, and that the disclosure of information should be restricted to achieve this purpose
- should document any disclosure of information, e.g.

  - the reasons for the disclosure
  - the content/extent of the disclosure
  - the person that authorised the disclosure

- must declare and ensure that signatories to the information-sharing partnership agreement are in full compliance with the common law duty of confidentiality and the standards set out by the Data Protection Act 1998 and the Caldicott Report, e.g.:

  - the information is only used for the purpose it was disclosed for, is retained safely and not for longer than necessary and is adequately destroyed
  - only the minimum necessary information should be shared
  - consent should be obtained if personal information is used/disclosed unless exceptional circumstances apply that permit the disclosure without consent
  - the data subject has a right of access to his/her data
  - the protection of third-party rights is guaranteed.

Health and Social Care Act 2001, section 60[6]

Section 60 of the Health and Social Care Act 2001 gives the Secretary of State the power to make orders that justify the disclosure and use of patient-identifiable and confidential information, even though the common law duty of confidentiality has not been satisfied in respect of this data. Although the disclosure of the confidential, patient-identifiable information under section 60 of the Health and Social Care Act constitutes a requirement of the law, the Data Protection Act 1998 continues to apply. It is therefore not enough just to rely on this exemption and not to give the patient fair processing information as this would be inconsistent with the disclosure. (Example: regulations under section 60 of the Health and Social Care Act require the GP to report a patient's diagnosed cancer to a cancer register. The GP continues to have the duty to inform the patient of the disclosure of his/her information and its consequences even though the clinician did not require the patient's consent for this disclosure.)[1]

The Secretary of State should consult with the independent statutory Patient Information Advisory Group (PIAG)[7] – which has the responsibility of representing the interest of those who would be affected by the regulations – before making any regulations under section 60 of the Health and Social Care Act. In those cases, where under this legislation confidential patient information is intended to be used or processed, additional safeguards and restrictions on the use and disclosure will apply to such information. These safeguards and restrictions might differ as each case will be looked at on its own merits and will be reviewed annually.

Section 60 of the Health and Social Care Act 2001 will lose its importance with the increasing availability of measures that allow either (through privacy-enhancing technology) patient confidential information to be more effectively anonymised or the appropriate recording of consent.

Freedom of Information Act 2000[8]

The Freedom of Information Act 2000 (FoI) gives individuals rights of access to information held by public authorities and those providing services for them.[9] FoI has been implemented in stages until January 2005. The reason for the staged implementation is to give those who are affected by this Act the chance to pre-pare for their new responsibilities. The Information Commissioner will oversee the implementation of the Act since both the Data Protection Act and the FoI Act regulate the handling of information.

The Information Commissioner has published guidance and interpretation of the FoI Act in June 2003, which will develop further, in particular through case law.

The FoI Act extends the individual's access rights under the Data Protection Act 1998 giving access to all types of information, whether personal or non-personal. Individuals will not be able to exercise their right of access until the body concerned has been phased in. Once this body has been phased in, the applicant will then have access to information recorded even before the Act was passed, unless any of the numerous exemptions of the Act apply and therefore the requested information does not need to be disclosed.

The FoI Act gives the individual the right

- to be told whether the information exists
- to receive that information.

The FoI Act strengthens the public's right to transparency and openness of public services and since the NHS and PHCTs provide a 'public service', they are covered by this Act. It is therefore the duty of the PHCT to ensure that people are aware of

- what information is available from the PHCT
- where to get hold of the information
- proposals for future service changes, reasons for it, the opportunity to influence these proposals or decisions
- explanations on decisions and actions taken with regard to their own treatment
- what services the PHCT is providing, how these are performing against locally and nationally set targets, if quality standards for these services are achieved, and their cost and effectiveness.

Responsibilities of the general medical practitioner[10]

- Identify a person (e.g. Caldicott Guardian/information governance lead/practice manager/GP) who will take on the responsibility of a Freedom of Information

lead (FoI lead) for the PHCT. This person should have similar person specifications as described in Chapter 1, Section 1, Caldicott Guardian/information governance lead.
- The FoI lead should receive adequate training.
- The name of the FoI lead should be published so that individuals know whom to ask for information.

Responsibilities of the FoI lead

- To ensure that the PHCT complies with the FoI Act.
- To develop and maintain a publication scheme (details of which are provided below).
- To ensure that individuals know what information is available from the PHCT.
- To respond to an individual's request for that information, either in providing that information or giving reasons for not disclosing that information if any exemption of the FoI Act applies.
- To ensure that the PHCT has got a clear and effective suggestions and complaints system.
- To ensure that individuals know how to get access to personal health records (which is regulated by the Data Protection Act 1998 and for deceased patients the Access to Health Records Act 1990).

Dealing with a request for information

- The individual requesting information does not need to give a reason for that request.
- The request can be in any form of writing giving the details of what is requested, name and address for correspondence and being capable to be used for future reference.
- Acknowledgement of the receipt of the request for information has to be given within four working days and the information should be provided not later than 20 working days unless certain exemptions apply.[11]
- In certain exceptional circumstances the applicant may be charged.[12]

Refusing a request: exemptions[13]

- In circumstances in which an exemption applies and the PHCT does not disclose the requested information, the applicant for this information should receive the reasons in writing within 20 working days from the date the information was requested.[14]
- The possibility that the released information may cause embarrassment or even loss of confidence in the PHCT or NHS or may be misunderstood is not necessarily a reason to refuse a request.[15]
- The PHCT is not required to make available copies of the documents or records that contain the information, or any information that already is widely in the public domain.[16]

- The PHCT is not required to provide information that it does not possess, i.e. it need not acquire any outside information for the applicant.
- Absolute exemptions apply to personal information[17] and information provided in confidence.[18] The Data Protection Act regulates the individual's right of access to their own health records which is not regulated under the FoI Act. The PHCT is bound under the common law duty of confidentiality to keep third-party information confidential unless the public interest outweighs the obligation to confidentiality.
- Among the qualified exemptions in the FoI Act, i.e. the certain circumstances under which information may be withheld are:

  - information (e.g. research) that is intended to be published in the future or prevents the holder from publishing it first[19]
  - information that may prejudice the outcome of legal proceedings or other legal matters[20]
  - information that may prejudice the outcome of negotiations or any contractual activities that are not internal NHS contracts[21]
  - information that is too difficult to provide because the request is too general or would require an unreasonable amount of resources.[22]

PHCT's publication schemes

The FoI Act requires every PHCT to establish its own publication scheme by January 2005 which should serve the following functions:

- provide a guide to all the information the PHCT is publishing or intends to publish
- give details of the services the PHCT provides
- provide assistance to people who would like to use their right of access to information e.g. in formulating a request.

The publication scheme has to be maintained, reviewed and updated and the scheme should be approved by the Commissioner. For medical practitioners the Commissioner has approved a model publication scheme that, if adopted by the PHCT, does not need to seek approval again. However, if the model publication scheme is modified by a PHCT, e.g. to be tailored to specific or local needs, then approval by the Commissioner is required.

Items that should form part of every PHCT's publication scheme are:[10]

- practice leaflets, which should contain the following essential information:

  - general practitioner(s): name, sex, qualifications, date and first place of registration and whether the GP works alone, part time or has partnership arrangements
  - clinics: purpose, frequency and duration
  - services provided by the PHCT, e.g. child health surveillance, contraception, maternity, minor surgery, counselling, anticoagulation treatment, physiotherapy, chiropody etc.
  - employed staff: numbers and roles (registration status)

  – repeat prescription and dispensing arrangements
  – boundary of geographical area which the practice is covering
  – information on access for the disabled
  – details on how suggestions, comments and complaints are handled

- plans of any changes in purchasing services
- plans on how the practice intends to use its funds, especially in view of achieving national and local targets
- annual reports on the PHCT's performance on GMS (General Medical Services) and PMS (Personal Medical Services) contracts as well as other national and local targets, e.g. from national service frameworks (NSFs), National Institute for Clinical Excellence (NICE) guidance etc.
- audited annual accounts: GPs will have to produce annual accounts for audit, after which these audited accounts are public documents.

Access to Health Records Act 1990[23]

The Access to Health Records Act 1990 regulates the access to deceased persons' records. Otherwise this Act has been largely superseded by the Data Protection Act 1998. Access to health records by living individuals is now regulated by the Data Protection Act 1998.

Computer Misuse Act 1990

The Computer Misuse Act 1990 makes unauthorised access or damage or modification to computerised information a criminal offence. This Act applies to any computer program or data, i.e. not just sensitive medical or person-identifiable data.

The following are important applications of the Computer Misuse Act for a PHCT:

- The sharing of passwords may provide the grounds for someone to gain unauthorised access. This constitutes a disciplinary offence.
- The authorisation to access computer material may be limited to the use of certain programs and data. Any use beyond that permission constitutes a criminal offence and therefore may provide the grounds for disciplinary proceedings.
- Any unauthorised modification of a computer program or data is a criminal offence. Every member of staff should be certain that any alterations (data entry, deletion) of a patient computer record are performed because of the duty or are otherwise authorised.

Copyright, Designs and Patents Act 1988

This Act aims to ensure that all intellectual works are treated on the same basis. The Act protects anything that has been created by someone from being copied or used by someone else without the payment to the originator. Computer programs are therefore protected by this Act. The person (or company) who has written the software is normally regarded as the holder of the copyright. Not only the copying but also the use of a computer program without the consent of the copyright owner is an infringement of the Act.

The PHCT will need to ensure that every member of staff complies with the law on licensed products and has to ensure that only licensed copies of software are used.

Public Interest Disclosure Act 1998

The Public Interest Disclosure Act 1998 updates part IV of the Employment Rights Act 1996. It establishes the concept of 'protected disclosure', which it defines as circumstances in which the employee reasonably believes that the disclosure is for the following reasons:

- a criminal offence has been or is likely to be committed
- a person has failed, is failing or is likely to fail to comply with any legal obligation
- a miscarriage of justice has occurred, is occurring or is likely to occur
- the health or safety of an individual has been, is being or is likely to be endangered
- the environment has been, is being or is likely to be damaged.

A disclosure of information is not a qualified disclosure if the person making the disclosure commits an offence by making it or if it is not done in good faith.

Children's Act 1989

Sections 17, 27, 47 and schedule 2 of the Children's Act 1989 provide statutory provisions that permit the sharing of information with regard to children and young people.

Section 17(1) requires every local authority to safeguard and promote the welfare of children.

Section 27 stipulates circumstances in which a local authority may request help from another authority. An authority (including health authority) whose help is so requested shall comply with the request if it is compatible with their own statutory or other duties and obligations and does not unduly prejudice the discharge of any of their functions.

Section 47 details the local authority's duty to investigate. Where local authorities are conducting enquiries under this section, it is the duty of any health authority to assist them with those enquiries, in particular by providing relevant information and advice.

Schedule 2 covers the prevention of neglect and abuse of children. It is the duty of every local authority to take reasonable steps, through the provision of services under part III of this Act, to prevent children within their area suffering ill-treatment or neglect. Where a local authority believes that a child who is at any time within their area and is likely to suffer harm, but lives in the area of another local authority, they shall inform that other local authority. When informing that other local authority they shall specify the harm that they believe the child is likely to suffer, and if possible where the child lives or proposes to live.

References

1   Information Commissioner (2002) *Use and Disclosure of Health Data: guidance on the application of the Data Protection Act 1998*, May.

2   *See* e.g. Data Protection Act 1998; section 60 of the Health and Social Act 2001.

3   The GMC's booklet *Confidentiality*, an associated leaflet to *Good Medical Practice*, gives guidance for health professionals on confidentiality and disclosure after a patient's death.

4   Human Rights Act: http://www.hmso.gov.uk/acts/acts/1998/19980042. htm.

5   Section 115 of the Crime and Disorder Act 1998.

6   Health and Social Care Act: http://www.hmso.gov.uk/acts/acts2001/2001 0015.htm. Only applicable in England and Wales.

7   Section 61 of the Health and Social Care Act 2001. Only applicable in England and Wales.

8   Freedom of Information Act: http://www.hmso.gov.uk/acts/acts2000/2000 00036.htm and http://www.informationcommissioner.gov.uk.

9   Information is defined in Freedom of Information Act 2000, Section 84.

10   DoH (1999) *Code of Practice on Openness in the NHS*.

11   Freedom of Information Act 2000, section 10(1). This is different from the requirement of the Data Protection Act 1998 which allows a response to be not later than 40 days after the receipt of the request: http://www.hmso.gov. uk/acts/acts2000/200000036.htm.

12   Freedom of Information Act 2000, section 9: http://www.hmso.gov.uk/acts/ acts2000/200000036.htm.

13   Part II of the Freedom of Information Act (sections 21 to 44).

14   Freedom of Information Act 2000, section 1(1)(a).

15   Information Commissioner (2003) *The Freedom of Information Act 2000: an introduction*, June. http://www.informationcommissioner.gov.uk

16   Freedom of Information Act 2000, section 21.

17   Freedom of Information Act 2000, section 40.

18   Freedom of Information Act 2000, section 41.

19   Freedom of Information Act 2000, section 22.

20   Freedom of Information Act 2000, sections 30 and 31.

21   Freedom of Information Act 2000, section 43.

22   Freedom of Information Act 2000, section 17.

23   Access to Health Records Act 1990: http://www.hmso.gov.uk/acts/acts/ 1990/Ukpga_19900023_en_1.htm.

Part Two

Christine Dainty

Chapter 4

Applying Caldicott to general practice

Introduction

The purpose of this chapter is to look at common scenarios found in general practice and to apply aspects of confidentiality and Caldicott Principles to those situations. There are no right or wrong answers. The scenario can be used either as a team exercise or on an individual basis.

The scenarios are fictional but based on true situations that have occurred in general practice. Questions posed are to stimulate your thoughts into a variety of areas that may be covered in each scenario. A description is given to each of the scenarios to expand the discussions you may have already had.

Each scenario is designed to bring out one or two particular aspects relating to confidentiality but you will find there are overbridging themes in many of them. The team or individual may prefer to expand the scenarios or create their own to form complex situations and enhance the discussion process.

Specific reference is made to sections in the Caldicott manual and additional references given as appropriate.

The area of confidentiality is constantly changing and therefore the interpretation is under constant review. The Caldicott lead for the practice and PCO will act as a valuable resource for PHCTs who wish to extend their knowledge in this area. The exercises may highlight additional training needs in the form of IT and communication skills for many staff dealing with the public.

Information for patients

Mr Black is 52 years old and was diagnosed with diabetes 12 months ago. He has been attending the local British Diabetic Association meeting held at the local hospital on a regular basis. Last night the meeting was attended by the local consultant providing diabetes care to the majority of diabetic patients in the area, including Mr Black. The topic for discussion was the use of the local diabetes register and how local GPs had made this successful, by being the main contributors of information from their registered diabetic patient records.

Mr Black arrives in surgery the next morning demanding to know what personal information has been released from the practice.

Questions to consider

1 What steps should the receptionist take with this patient?
2 How has the Data Protection Act been applied?
3 What mechanisms does the practice have for informing patients of the use of information about patients?
4 Who has obtained consent and to what has the patient consented?

Points for discussion

Practice complaints procedure

Front-line staff are often the first to encounter a patient's complaint about the services within a practice or an aspect of their healthcare. Staff should all undergo training in communications skills including verbal de-escalation skills. Sensitive handling of the patient at this stage may diffuse any further complaints. Listening to the patient's concerns and answering any questions regarding the confidential aspects of his care may be all the patient needs. Additional information may be required from the practice manager to further reassure the patient.

The patient may wish to pursue this complaint through the practice complaints procedure and put his concerns in writing to the practice. The receptionist should be able to provide the patient with the nominated person in the practice (usually the practice manager) who will deal with his complaint.

A polite approach towards the patient often helps reduce the level of aggression during such discussions. Patients who are verbally or physically abusive or threatening should be instructed of the zero tolerance approach taken by the practice. A notice in reception or public areas of the practice will advertise the practice's philosophy on this issue. Further reinforcement in the practice leaflet or website is useful.

Data protection act

Medical information about a patient cannot be released from the practice without the patient's consent. The practice also has a legal responsibility to keep personal-identifiable information about a patient confidential. Releasing anonymised data in the form of audits is widespread and they are an invaluable tool in improving the quality of care. Often audits are done within the practice, as part of PCO activity, regionally or even nationally based. Such activities are an essential part of monitoring the standards of care delivered to the local population and also in the planning and commissioning of services for the local population.

Local diabetes registers often contain identifiable information and therefore require the consent of the patient. Clarification of what information was gathered and presented in the meeting is relevant to the perceived breach of trust by the patient.

Practice leaflets and posters

Under the requirements of Caldicott, patients need to be informed about the use of their confidential information.

Posters in the waiting room and written information in leaflets or the practice leaflet will enable patients to be informed of the uses of patients' information, e.g. delivering services locally. The information should be explicit so patients are fully informed.

Informed consent

Doctors are required to ensure that patients fully understand the term informed consent. It is not adequate that patients give verbal consent or written consent without an explanation of what information will be disclosed or the purpose of the disclosure* (*see* Chapter 1, Section 5, and Chapter 2).

Patients attending the diabetes clinic should be counselled by the practice nurse to obtain their consent for inclusion of their data onto the local diabetes register. Some practice nurses and GPs may be well versed in obtaining written consent from their patients for this type of activity. This type of consent may well apply to other clinical areas.

Summary

1   Practice complaints policy (*see* Chapter 6) and NHS complaints procedure (*see* Chapter 5).
2   Data Protection Act 1998: http://www.legislation.hmso.gov.uk.
3   Practice leaflets for informing patients (*see* Chapter 1, Section 5).
4   Informed consent and consent forms (*see* Chapter 1, Section 5, and Chapter 2).

Staff conduct and patient confidentiality

> Betty has worked as a practice nurse for several years in a single-handed practice. She is prone to gossip about patients but never discloses any names. On one occasion she discusses openly with other members of staff in the practice how a patient had contracted hepatitis B from a prostitute while on holiday abroad. The patient's name is mentioned in the details.

Questions to consider

1   If this comes to the notice of her employers, what action, if any, should they take?
2   What aspects regarding staff contracts need to be discussed and why?
3   What is the role of the Caldicott Guardian in this case?

Points for discussion

1   Staff code of conduct.
2   Contract of employment.
3   Professional responsibilities.
4   Roles and responsibilities of the Caldicott Guardian.
5   Practice induction and training programme.

---

* General Medical Council (2004) *Confidentiality: protecting and providing information.* GMC, London.

1   Staff code of conduct (*see* Chapter 1, Section 2).
2   The contract of employment should contain a term relating to breaches of
    confidentiality and how the employer would respond (*see* Chapter 1, Section 6).
        Staff should appreciate that disclosure of patient information in unjustified
    circumstances is a serious disciplinary offence for which action will be taken by
    employers (http://www.doh.gov.uk/confiden/index.htm).
3   She may be reported to her professional body – the Nursing and Midwifery
    Council (www.nmc-uk.org).
4   For the roles and responsibilities of the Caldicott Guardian within the practice
    in relation to staff training *see* Section 20, Implementation strategy, points 2, 4,
    5, 7, 8 and 12.
5   For the practice induction and training programme relating to confidentiality
    see Chapter 1, Section 3.

Staff induction and training

Susie has just been appointed by the practice as a new member of office staff.
She has had six months' experience in a large inner-city practice. Her duties
will involve mostly filing, general office duties and dealing with prescriptions. The office supervisor has been given the task of staff induction.

Questions to consider

1   Who is responsible for her training?
2   What areas should be covered during her induction procedure and why?
3   How can you ensure all the training needs have been covered?
4   What tools can be used to ensure regular confidentiality training?

Points for discussion

Responsibility for training

Staff will require training appropriate to their grade and job description and also
according to the duties the employers expect of them. Most GPs employ a
practice manager who will carry the responsibility of training new staff during an
induction period. Practices will vary in their approach depending on the employee
and resources available to them. Many practices undertake a formal induction
phase with supplementary in-house supervision and training. Practices may be able
to approach PCOs who often employ IT trainers to enable new staff to grasp the
technology within the practice.
    The Caldicott Guardian should also ensure that adequate confidentiality and
Caldicott issues are covered in this phase.

Staff code of conduct

Individuals entering employment with the NHS come from a variety of sources
and backgrounds. It should not be assumed that they are familiar with the high

standards of conduct expected when dealing with the public and dealing with confidential issues. Organisations have to be explicit to employees what is expected of them in their duties.

Data Protection Act
All individuals must have a basic understanding of the Data Protection Act and how it should be interpreted within their sphere of work. The organisation has a responsibility to ensure that staff handling confidential and sensitive information treat this information in an appropriate manner.

Caldicott Principles
A general understanding of the principles (*see* Chapter 1, Caldicott Principles) is important so employees can appreciate the need to treat patient-identifiable information as importantly as most healthcare professionals. An explanation of how the principles apply to the duties individuals perform can reinforce this concept. Specific training may be required for use of the fax machine (safe haven) and security access to the clinical system used in the practice. PCOs may provide learning events related to confidentiality and Caldicott issues.

IM&T training
Most practices are moving away from paper records towards electronic patient records. Most employees including the PHCT will require a range of computing skills to enable them to perform their duties and record a range of information required for patient care. Training is often ongoing and supported by a variety of specific trainers in the clinical systems in common use.

Some individuals may already have a degree of computing skills when starting with a new practice. The induction period is an opportunity to identify the strengths of the individual's computer skills as well as gaps in skills and knowledge. Due to the varied range of expertise required in IT skills it may be beneficial to the practice to have several individuals trained to various levels of expertise.

Security policy and training responsibilities
Specific user names are given to individuals using the clinical system in the practice together with a unique password, which should only be used by the individual. User names and passwords act as a 'signature' when logged into the system. This will result in an electronic audit trail. This tool can be invaluable when investigating perceived errors. Practical steps such as logging in, logging off, and locking computers away when unattended are simple measures to reduce the risk of security breaches.

Safe havens
This refers to the use of fax machines. A full description is given in the scenario Safe haven.

Procedure checklist
To ensure each individual receives a basic and comprehensive coverage of essential issues relating to confidentiality a checklist is a useful tool. It can enable the assessor to cover quickly all the areas required and identify gaps in a consistent

manner, and subsequent reviews will show successive improvements in those areas. A checklist is provided in Chapter 1, Section 3, Staff induction procedures.

Regular appraisal/annual updating of confidentiality and security issues
Most employees within the NHS expect an annual appraisal by a senior colleague or line manager. This is an opportunity to obtain feedback on performance and to identify continual professional development. Issues relating to confidentiality and Caldicott are complex and continually changing. Staff and the PHCT will need to have regular updates on new developments in legislation and interpretation of regulations governing access and confidentiality.

Summary

1   Staff code of conduct (*see* Chapter 1, Section 2).
2   Principles of Data Protection Act 1998 (*see* Chapter 2) (http://www.legisla tion.hmso.gov.uk).
3   Caldicott Principles (*see* Chapter 1).
4   IM&T training provision (*see* Chapter 1, Section 4).
5   Security policy and user responsibilities (*see* Chapter 1, Sections 12, 17 and 18).
6   Security responsibilities (*see* Chapter 1, Section 13).
7   Safe-haven procedures – fax machine (*see* Chapter 1, Section 10).
8   Procedure checklist (*see* Chapter 1, Section 4).
9   Regular appraisal/annual updating of confidentiality and security issues.

Confidentiality agreements

There is building work being undertaken at Practice B and this involves workmen accessing the reception area. As you walk through to collect some notes you notice that a number of referral letters are waiting to be signed. You then become aware of patients' notes, appointment books and blood results, which are all clearly visible.

Questions to consider

1   What confidentiality aspects are being breached?
2   How does the Data Protection Act apply here?
3   Which additional tool could be used to maintain confidentiality?

Points for discussion

Breaches in confidentiality
A variety of individuals have access to practice premises, who are not necessarily employed by the practice. Visitors may include patients, employees of the PCO, colleagues from neighbouring practices, contract cleaners, workmen, communication engineers etc.

Simple measures can be very effective in reducing the risk of breaching confidentiality. Where possible individual case notes should be filed away promptly and not left in public areas or on display where the public may see them.

All reception staff through induction training should be made aware of the confidential aspect of medical records and personal data in the form of names and addresses on the front of medical notes and letters.

Letters and laboratory results could be left in designated areas away from public view, e.g. in folders for the doctor or nurse to review or sign.

Electronic records remove a large amount of the physical requirement of paper notes and hence reduce the overall risk of unauthorised access. Electronic records restrict casual access to patient notes due to the security access that is required (*see* Chapter 1, Section 4).

Data Protection Act

The Data Protection Act indicates the level of responsibility to which organisations are held accountable to safeguard the personal information held within their files. Medical information requires a greater degree of confidentiality due to the sensitive nature of the information held.

The responsibility for protecting all aspects of personal data lies with the individual practice. Although the practice is not intentionally releasing patient information, there are a range of measures that could be used to improve this confidentiality (*see* Chapter 2, Data Protection Act).

Confidentiality agreements

Staff members should have, within their contract of employment, a clear statement regarding confidentiality, in relation to the information they handle in the practice. The practice should make it very clear to prospective employees the obligations of their duties and aspects of confidentiality and the seriousness of breaches of confidentiality. Often the contract will make specific details regarding disciplinary procedures and possible dismissal depending on the seriousness of breaching confidentiality.

Confidentiality agreements can also be used for outside agencies and contractors who have access to the practice, either on a regular basis or an ad hoc basis. This either has to be part of the agency's contract or the practice will have to ask the agency employee to sign a confidentiality agreement (*see* Chapter 1, Section 7).

Summary

(Relevant sections in the Caldicott manual are indicated in brackets.)

1   Confidentiality and training needs (*see* Chapter 1, Section 4).
2   Data Protection Principles (*see* Chapter 2).
3   Confidentiality agreements (*see* Chapter 1, Section 7).

Also consider:

4   Information flows (*see* Chapter 1, Section 8).
5   Safe-haven procedures (*see* Chapter 1, Section 10).

Data ownership

A social worker contacts the surgery saying that a member of the public has contacted the duty office with concerns over a neighbour. After accessing the property it appears that the patient has been neglecting himself for a number of months, and the social worker suspects alcohol to be the underlying cause. The social worker can take steps to put in care for the patient but he needs the information faxing over this afternoon to enable the situation to be sorted out today for the benefit of all concerned. As the GP you are also aware that the patient suffers from a significant personality disorder and often is abusive and refuses help.

Questions to consider

1   How does the Data Protection Act apply to this case?
2   What protocols are in place governing the sharing of patient information?
3   What Caldicott Principles apply?
4   Who owns the information?
5   What measures are taken to keep the information safe?
6   How will the data be used?

Points for discussion

Data Protection Act

This is not an uncommon situation in general practice, often involving a third party requesting information about a patient registered at the practice.

Information that identifies the individual is also covered by this Act. The information held within the medical record is protected under the Data Protection Act and under patient confidentiality.

The practice staff should seek advice from either the Caldicott Guardian within the practice or the doctor concerned with the patient's medical treatment. Consent is required from the patient for release of medical information. Although the patient may not have given written consent, verbal consent may be obtained from the patient regarding passing relevant information to the social worker.

Protocols for sharing information

Dealing with such a request highlights the need for the practice to have an understanding of the process of dealing with access to patient information. The practice should have a clear process in place, which members of the PHCT can follow, when outside agencies request information regarding a patient registered at the practice.

Not only is access to the patient's information restricted to outside agencies but clinical data may be restricted to members of the PHCT, depending on their individual security access level. Information held within the patient's medical records is only shared with other members of the team on a need-to-know basis. Usually information is shared between the PHCT to enhance the care provided for the patient.

Caldicott Principles

There is an implied trust that the social worker will use this data to enhance the care provision for the patient and that the doctor is acting in the best interests of the patient. Ultimately, the clinician will be faced with the decision of whether confidential information regarding this patient needs to be disclosed. Which information needs to be disclosed is also relevant. The clinician may decide that maintaining confidentiality overrides all other aspects of the patient's care.

Often multidisciplinary teams have to share a degree of knowledge about a patient, so that each member of the team can provide the aspect of medical/nursing/social care required from the team member. If there remains any doubt over the decision to release information then advice should be sought from the medical defence organisation used by the practice.

Any information released will be on a 'need-to-know' basis. It would be inappropriate to release information of a sensitive nature not relevant to the patient's needs at this time. It would be helpful if the social worker could specify what information is required, preferably in writing, e.g. via fax machine.

Ownership and control of data

Theoretically the data is owned by the patient. For practical purposes the 'owner' is often the GP involved with the patient's care. Other health professionals, e.g. district nurses, hold their own separate confidential notes on the patients. A Caldicott lead within the practice can provide guidance on what information can be released. Further advice can be obtained from the PCO Caldicott lead.

If the decision has been made that relevant information can be released, provision must be made to ensure that information is transferred securely. While email is still uncommon, there needs to be in place a clear policy in the practice regarding external emails containing sensitive information, possibly including encryption.

Faxes are often a convenient way of transmitting information quickly. Steps must be taken by the practice to ensure that the information transmitted will only be viewed by those who need to see it (safe haven, *see* Chapter 1, Section 10).

Alternatively, the GP may wish to visit the patient and access the situation independently, involving social services as appropriate.

Summary

(Relevant sections in the Caldicott manual are indicated in brackets.)

1   Data Protection Act (*see* Chapter 2)
2   Caldicott Principles (*see* Chapter 1).
3   Agreeing who is allowed to have access to this confidential data (*see* Chapter 1, Section 18).
    Securing data.
    How the data will be used when determining the sensitivity of it (*see* Chapter 1, Section 9).
4   Safe-haven procedures (*see* Chapter 1, Section 10).
5   Protocols to govern information sharing (*see* Chapter 1, Section 11).

Safe haven

The practice has only one fax machine.

Thursdays is half day at the practice and the practice is closed. A fax was sent to the practice at 4.00 pm from the local hospital. It contained patient-identifiable information and a clinical diagnosis of an advanced brain tumour.

One of the people with access to the room early the next morning was a clinical waste collector. He reads the fax, as his company had indicated to him that they would be contacting the practice to enquire about his collection times and therefore he thought the fax was relating to this.

Questions to consider

1   What is a security incident and how are they monitored?
2   What protocols does the practice have for sharing information?
3   What safety measures are taken with outside contractors?
4   How are information flows reviewed?
5   What is meant by a safe haven?

Points for discussion

Monitoring security incidents

Unfortunately confidentiality has been breached. It is essential to determine the details of this incident to prevent future similar incidents. Human error does occur and this may have been an isolated event. The contractor may well have worked in the practice long term and used this method of communicating with his firm before. Since this incident, it may be more appropriate for the company to ring the employee instead.

There may have been a valid reason for the contractor to be in the office as part of his duties. Consider other individuals who may be in the office as part of their duties and may be exposed to a similar situation.

Security breaches may be monitored as they occur and the situation leading to them reviewed to prevent future occurrences. Proactive steps may be adopted by reviewing aspects of practice and highlighting areas causing concern. Specific steps can then be discussed and implemented as part of a risk management approach.

Protocols governing the sharing of information

The onus is on the practice to ensure that the fax machine is in a secure place. An upstairs locked office restricts access to those individuals who have security access to both the fax machine and office.

The practice must ensure that information faxed into the practice is only accessed by those involved with the patient's care on a need-to-know basis.

Therefore placing the fax machine in an area that very few people access for other reasons reduces the risk of unauthorised access.

Contracts with outside organisations

Practices must ensure that contracts placed with an outside contractor contain a clause pertaining to confidentiality. While most firms working with the NHS appreciate the sensitivity of information that their employees come into contact with, as employers they must maintain the same high standards that are seen within the NHS. If the contract does not contain a clause, then a confidentiality agreement must be signed by the contractor's employee.

Confidentiality agreements

Most practices will appreciate that employees are exposed to confidential information about patients on a regular basis. Usually a clause in the employment contract will recognise the importance of maintaining confidentiality and the seriousness of disclosure. Some employers will insist on a signed confidentiality agreement.

Practices may insist on visitors signing confidentiality agreements. This would include outside contractors or agencies who come into the practice on a regular or ad hoc basis.

Information flows

Most written material held within a record can be linked to an individual by their name, address or date of birth. This is the commonest method of identifying patients registered on a practice's list. Any faxed material usually carries the same identifiable information.

Using an individual's NHS number, which is not commonly known to the general public, can be an alternative method to identify an individual. This will significantly reduce the risk of others knowing the patient's identity (*see* Chapter 1, Section 8, Reviewing information flows).

Safe-haven procedures

Fax machines have become a valuable method of communication. Faxed information into a practice can provide immediate and necessary details about a patient's condition or aspect of their care. Similarly it can be an explicit means of providing specific information about a patient to a third party, e.g. rapid access referrals for suspected cancers.

Fax machines should be regarded with care because of patient confidentiality and the sensitive written information faxes may contain. Machines should ideally be placed out of public view. If possible, machines could be placed in a more secure part of the building, e.g. in an office manned by practice staff, reducing the risk of unauthorised access.

A notice placed on the door of the office in which the fax machine is housed stating 'safe haven' can also alert those entering the room of the presence of sensitive material.

A copy of the Caldicott Principles on the wall next to the fax machine can be a useful reminder to staff that they have thought about the justification of exchanging information.

A confidential header on information faxed out of the practice can warn the recipient of the sensitive nature of the information. It may also alert individuals that information being transmitted is not authorised for their access.

Information requested from an outside agency must contain an organisation letter-head, to reduce the risk of unauthorised access.

Summary

(Relevant sections in the Caldicott manual are indicated in brackets.)

1   Security incidents and monitoring (*see* Chapter 1, Sections 15 and 16).
2   Protocols governing sharing of information (*see* Chapter 1, Section 11).
3   Contracts placed with other organisations (*see* Chapter 1, Section 7).
4   Confidentiality agreements for visitors.
5   Information flows (*see* Chapter 1, Section 8).
6   Safe-haven procedures (*see* Chapter 1, Section 10).

Security monitoring

Mary has worked as a receptionist at the practice for one year. She works on reception dealing with enquiries and appointments. One of her new duties is to issue repeat prescriptions. On a very busy day her colleague Denise offered to help her process the repeat prescriptions. Denise logged onto the computer using her password.

The following month a patient requested a repeat prescription for a certain medication. The computer showed up a hazard warning and the receptionist informed the patient that they should not be taking that particular drug. The patient was very upset and worried because they had been taking it for a month and made a written complaint.

The practice manager conducted an investigation into the complaint. The audit trail showed that Denise, the head receptionist, had issued the drug as her password was shown on the script issued.

Questions to consider

1   How would you determine what has happened with this prescription error?
2   What access controls are currently in place to prevent unauthorised access to the computer's clinical system?
3   What information and training have the staff received in regard to performing their duties in the practice?
4   How are such incidents monitored and lessons learnt from them?
5   What training should staff receive to prevent such incidents occurring in the future?
    What tools are available to help identify the learner's needs?
6   Who is responsible for this breach?

Points for discussion

Prescription errors are common and are thought to occur in approximately 10% of prescriptions issued. It is essential staff are adequately trained to perform the duties that are required of them. Additional information on repeat prescribing can be found in the office policy section in Chapter 6. There is also an audit tool to assist practices to review the repeat prescribing policy currently used. This audit can be found in the Appendix on p. 187. For more information on the prescribing audits please contact graham.pimblett@southsefton-pct.nhs.uk.

Determining what has happened

An investigation of this incident highlights the importance of the electronic audit trail and the identification of the individual responsible for the mistake. Using this example as a significant event analysis allows the PHCT to identify gaps in specific skills and further training provided to prevent similar episodes in the future. Clarification from both receptionists revealed that Denise had not logged out of the system. Work done by Mary had been logged under Denise's password. The need to log-out and protect personal passwords must be explained during staff induction and computer training.

Each member of staff must have a unique user name and password, which is only known to them. Every time a member of staff logs into the computer system an electronic audit trail is generated. This allows the practice to trace work done in the practice using the computer, e.g. issuing prescriptions, booking appointments. Staff should not tell each other their passwords for security reasons.

Staff code of conduct

All members of the PHCT must be aware of the basic Caldicott Principles with regard to patients' confidential material held in the patient's medical record and details identifying the patient. In addition individuals using a clinical system maintain individual user responsibility to prevent security breaches during their access of the computer system.

Various duties involving the computer system will require staff members to have different access levels to computer functions. Higher levels of access to computer functions are often associated with advanced computing and a greater degree of responsibility.

Practice security policies

Adequate induction procedures for new members of staff will help familiarise them with practice systems and practice policies. Separate computer training on a regular basis is essential to maintain high quality performance in general practice.

Most practices will be able to provide in-house training towards a basic level of computing skills. More complex skills may be required in only a small number of key personnel. Often PCOs will have personnel to help train staff to use specific computer systems.

Advanced IT training is usually provided by PCOs locally in the provision of IT trainers. The Caldicott Guardian may use the opportunity of such incidents to hold multidisciplinary team meetings and use the incident in a positive light, as a means of illustrating the importance of practice procedures.

Security monitoring

Monitoring can be done as specific breaches occur, usually highlighted as an incident occurring in the practice. Some may come to light as a result of a patient's complaint. Others may be brought to the attention of the practice manager or Caldicott Guardian by members of the PHCT as part of daily working.

Often significant event auditing, using a whole PHCT approach, can result in significant awareness raising within the team. Small changes can result in an improvement immediately towards achieving Caldicott compliance, e.g. not using each other's passwords.

Alternatively the practice may wish to conduct audits in the practice, on a regular basis. Specific areas could be looked at, over the long term, to measure what improvements have taken place, e.g. safe-haven procedures.

Security training updates

Regular staff appraisal by a senior colleague should help individuals identify their learning needs in a variety of areas. Often individuals are aware of gaps in their skills and use the appraisal process to identify resources to provide further training. Experienced managers often use appraisals to give constructive feedback to employees on their strengths and learning needs in the performance of their duties.

During individual assessments a template or tick box can aid full coverage of IT training (*see* Chapter 1, Section 4). This will ensure comprehensive coverage of all aspects of confidentiality that personnel may require. PCOs may have adopted specific training requirements for practices to enhance standardisation and consistency of approach towards confidentiality issues.

Security responsibilities

Everyone is responsible for security of data confidentiality. Each member of the team holds an important position in ensuring systems run efficiently in the practice. Each individual holds responsibility for accessing the computer, maintaining personal passwords and logging out of systems when finished. Caldicott Guardians oversee the entire strategy for the practice and should strive towards excellence in the workplace and complying with all aspects of Caldicott, confidentiality and access.

Summary

(Relevant sections in the Caldicott manual are indicated in brackets.)

1 Staff code of conduct (*see* Chapter 1, Section 2).
2 Access responsibility and access control (*see* Chapter 1, Sections 17 and 18).
3 Practice protocols/security policies (*see* Chapter 1, Section 17).
4 Security monitoring (*see* Chapter 1, Section 16).
5 Security training update (*see* Chapter 1, Section 4).
6 Security responsibilities (*see* Chapter 1, Section 13).

Physical threats

> The practice manager rings you early Saturday morning to inform you that the practice has been vandalised overnight and it appears that some equipment is missing. It seems that a downstairs window was left open on the Friday evening. The police are at the surgery making a report but you will need to co-ordinate with the practice manager to make an inventory of what is missing and an assessment for the insurance company.

Questions to consider

1   Have you got an inventory of equipment?
2   How much is the value or importance of your equipment?
3   How would you measure the impact that this loss or destruction would cause?
4   Can you list these components and their value?
5   How vulnerable is your equipment, e.g. are items easily reached through an open window?
6   What is the risk regarding theft?
7   What is the risk of physical damage, e.g. fire, flood and vandalism?

Each of the above questions has to apply to every single item of the inventory.

Points for discussion

Inventory of equipment

Most practices do not realise the amount of equipment the practice holds on the premises, or the full impact of its loss, on the daily functioning of the practice. For large practices the list may be extensive and costly to replace.

A full list of equipment includes computer hardware in the form of:

* computer terminal(s)
* printer(s)
* scanner(s)
* keyboard(s)
* palmtop(s).

All these items have a monetary value and would probably require immediate replacement for the practice to function properly and efficiently. Practices that are paper light are especially vulnerable to loss of the above hardware, as the computer has become the physical means of recording the consultation and accessing patient notes. Other essential equipment includes:

* backup tapes/disks
* fax machine
* answerphone
* software
* paper records (files, letters, incoming and outgoing post).

Practices may also have on site a video recording machine, video camera and television, which are often used for training purposes.

Assessing the value of equipment

Although an insurance company may acknowledge the financial cost of replacing equipment from an insurance claim, most professionals would recognise the impact that the loss or destruction would cause, in attempting to function as a practice without this equipment. Keeping written records rather than an electronic record can be difficult for clinicians who have become accustomed to paper-light systems. Booking appointments and issuing prescriptions may become a logistical impossibility for reception staff. Some thought of how the practice may overcome these difficulties is useful.

It may become apparent after the loss of essential equipment that immediate replacement is essential. There may be a delay in reimbursement from the insurance company. PCOs may be able to loan equipment or offer financial assistance in the short term. Consider how the practice could afford to replace the items in full from the practice account.

Risk of physical damage to equipment

Most buildings can act as a target for burglary. General practices may pose an additional attraction due to the storage of drugs and medical equipment.

Staff may be fully aware of the security access into the computer system through training but may not be aware of the vulnerability of equipment if left unattended. Ground floor offices are often more accessible than upper floors to open windows and opportunistic access.

Locks on doors are an effective way of preventing unauthorised access into areas of the practice that house expensive equipment.

Offices should be locked when empty, windows closed, window locks used if fitted, and alarms fitted and set – these can all help to reduce the risk of unauthorised access to the practice building. Regularly raising awareness helps individuals working in the practice recognise these possible threats before an incident occurs. Possible physical risks to consider are the risk of theft, fire, flood and vandalism.

Adequate fire prevention, smoke alarms, health and safety regulations and regular external inspection by either the Health and Safety Executive, local fire services or crime prevention services can provide useful advice to prevent future incidents. Risk assessments are a vital tool to assessing risk as well as rising awareness (*see* Chapter 1, Section 14).

Software and computer viruses

On arrival at surgery, you switch on the computer to check your emails. There appear to be several messages from outside your usual contacts. There has already been a message from the PCT warning users about computer viruses disrupting a local practice system for most of a working day.

Questions to consider

1 What is the possibility of a security threat, e.g. the threat regarding unauthorised use or modification of computers or the risk of viruses infecting the software and/or the risk of a program failing?
2 What is the risk of confidential information being disclosed that has not been authorised, e.g. are passwords being written down, making them accessible to other people?
3 What would the possible impact be if any security breach occurred with regard to the risk to:

   • the individual patient
   • the practice systems?

4   Which type of information would be:

- lost
- modified
- destroyed?

Points for discussion

Security threats

Computer viruses are commonplace and require most software to include an up-to-date virus checker. Virus infection can result from email transmission or using software that is infected. Infection from a virus can lead to severe disruption of software programs and disruption of the computer system in the practice. Although the equipment is still present, the inability to use a computer for daily activities and functioning of the practice will have an equivalent effect of physical loss of the equipment.

Unauthorised use or modification of computers, the risk of viruses infecting the software and/or the risk of a program failing can lead to the same frustrations as the equipment being stolen as described in the previous example.

Regulating updating the virus checker on the computer is essential. A degree of caution should be exercised when opening emails from an unknown source. Often PCOs or local practices send bulletins to neighbouring practices to warn of recent virus infection.

Training in confidentiality

Regular training of staff in the use of emails and having an email policy in place can help reduce the risk of opening emails infected with a virus.

Training of staff to use passwords will reduce the risk of access to the computer by non-authorised personnel. Passwords also prevent employees accessing a level of security that they are not authorised to access. Preventing access to the computer system blocks physical access to medical information and protects the confidentiality of the patient.

Screen savers used in the doctors' and nurses' consultation rooms prevent patients inadvertently observing other patients' medical details. The use of screen savers within reception areas may reduce the risk of the general public viewing information on the computer system.

Clear guidance should be given to staff on what information can be given under the Data Protection Act. Caldicott Guardians should provide an induction and training to staff regarding confidentiality in the practice. Regular training and confidentiality awareness-raising improves staff knowledge and reduces future breaches of unauthorised information.

Impact of security breaches

The individual patient

Most patients registered at a practice would probably not be aware that their notes are not accessible unless they attended the practice to see a health professional. Attendance by the patient at the practice on a day when the system is not functioning can be frustrating for both the patient and the doctor. Concerns for the doctor include consulting a patient with an incomplete medical record or who has been given a prescription for a known drug allergy.

Inability to access patient notes can affect a range of services that would normally be routine administrative tasks, e.g. call and recall systems, booking appointments, issuing prescriptions.

Unauthorised access by individuals within the practice and outside the practice could result in confidential information from medical notes being released without the patient's consent.

The practice systems

Corruption of the practice system can result in a difficult working environment for patients and staff. It can be costly in time, money and personnel to put the problem right. Usually expertise will be required to reinstate the computer programs. Often this expertise will not be found in the practice. PCOs or the computer software supplier may be able to offer advice.

Corruption of data

Information that is corrupted may result in information being lost, destroyed or modified. Depending on the level of disruption, material may be retrieved and reinstated in its original format. Although this may be costly and time consuming the alternative is permanent loss of data and information from the computer record. It is essential that electronic information is backed up from the computer on a regular basis, usually daily. Regular copying of files significantly reduces the loss of large amounts of electronic data. Copied files should be stored off site to prevent loss or damage through fire, flood, vandalism and theft.

Chapter 5

Practical aspects of confidentiality, Caldicott and access

Introduction

Confidentiality is a cornerstone of medical practice. Protecting the personal data of patients and handling medical information poses additional challenges for individuals working in general practice. While there is legislation and professional obligations to consider, NHS staff require guidance on how confidential information needs to be handled in a variety of common situations.

In addition individuals working within the NHS have to adapt to new technologies, contractual changes, service redesign and developments in working across organisation boundaries. While most professions will consider this to the benefit of the patient and the care they receive, there are also potential areas of concern to overcome.

The following chapter provides information on a range of common situations to be found in general practice. Scenarios are provided to help healthcare teams and individuals explore a range of issues relating to Caldicott and confidentiality. Chapter 6, on practice policies, provides a range of useful frameworks, applicable to practical situations within daily general practice work.

Confidentiality: NHS Code of Practice provides a useful guide to assist us in interpreting how patient information should be handled in the emerging new NHS.

Retention of records

A partner at the practice has decided to become a trainer for GP registrars. The partners agree to participate in adopting the standards required to become a training practice. The new computer system has vastly improved the quality of the summarising. During this process the partners are surprised at the amount of information and the age of some of the letters in the patients' paper records.

1   What constitutes a patient's record?
2   How long should records be kept?
3   When are electronic records deleted?

The patient record

Traditional practice involved paper records usually in the form of Lloyd George notes. Generally a patient's record would contain:

- written notes from the health professional involved with the patient's care
- correspondence from other healthcare professionals
- non-medical correspondence, e.g. insurance forms, correspondence from outside agencies regarding disability awards
- investigation results, e.g. x-rays, blood results.

Due to the increasing complexity of medical investigations, written patient records can become extremely bulky, with increasing difficulty in retrieving relevant information. Training practices were some of the first to adopt a system that requires patients' notes to be summarised and in date order. This facilitates the PHCT to access appropriate information to enhance the continuity of care for patients, as well as providing quality care. This approach also benefited the whole primary care team. Many non-training practices have adopted a similar standard.

Records maintaintence

The current recommendations from the DoH are that medical records should be maintained for certain periods of time (*see* retention of records in Chapter 1, Section 10).

There have been instances where cases have involved medical records dating long before the suggested length of retention.

Deletion of electronic records

General practice has also seen the introduction of computerised clinical systems, which have resulted in a growing number of practices becoming 'paper light'. The PHCT, are now familiar with entering information about patients, under clinical headings or Read codes, directly onto the patient's electronic record (PER). Paper documents in the form of letters from medical colleagues, patients, outside agencies and investigations can be scanned into the computer system for storage and incorporation into the clinical record.

GPs must not destroy or delete their electronic records until records can be transferable in their entirety (including the audit trail) between clinical systems.

In practical terms GPs are not required to delete the electronic records of ex-patients. Most clinical systems will allow the deducted patients' records to be hidden and only re-activated if the patients re-register at the practice.

Many practices have the additional burden of keeping manual records as well as electronic records during transitional phases, as practices become computerised. This system is often referred to as dual patient records.

Summary

Retention of records

- Retention of a patient's record varies according to the content and nature of the medical records. Do not assume all records are kept for the same time.
- A patient's record includes all written/electronic records, letters, laboratory investigations and reports.
- Paper and electronic records carry equal legal weight.
- Electronic records cannot at present be from a practice clinical system, due to difficulties in transferring the records from clinical systems between practices.
- Records need to kept in safe secure premises, including security measures for access to electronic records.
- Despite guidance on the length on the retention of records, there are a few medico-legal cases brought to light after an extensive period of time.

Further reading

HSC 1998/217: *Preservation, Retention and Destruction of GP General Medical Services Records Relating to Patients.*

Quality of record keeping

The PHCT based at the practice have taken several years to transfer from paper records to electronic patient records and now consider the practice 'paper light'. All the clinical staff have participated in additional training to make this transition successful. The team are now reviewing what additional benefits can be achieved by continuing to refine the electronic record.

---

1 What additional training is required for staff?
2 What additional benefits do electronic records bring?
3 What external resources are available to practices in electronic record keeping?

Training for staff

Accurate and legible medical notes are essential to good medical practice. Whether notes are kept in paper or electronic forms, practices are obliged to keep accurate records, which are legible, dated and recorded in a way that they cannot be erased or the original entry easily read. Logging in and out of the clinical system allows an electronic audit of data entered into the patient's notes, the date added and identification of the health professional accessing and updating the medical record. All the PHCT need to understand the importance of user names and passwords, which are unique to themselves.

Keeping comprehensive notes in an electronic form requires additional skills in documentation methods and keyboard skills. Further skills include the use of correct disease Read codes.

Additional benefits of electronic records

Accurate and well-structured notes assist the PHCT in accessing the correct information in a timely manner. Accessing quality data should enhance the quality of care provided to the patient and help reduce the risks associated with clinical practice, e.g. inappropriate drug prescribing, failure to monitor renal function in diuretic treatment. Use of Read codes among the PHCT allows for standardisation of diagnoses within the practice population.

The new GP contract will also result in a variety of standardised 'template' entries for a variety of chronic diseases, to obtain the maximum quality indicator scores.

This essential data is often used for clinical audit, clinical care of the patients, planning and commissioning for future services, both at practice and PCO levels, and clinical research. Therefore it is essential that this data is high quality and accurate.

External sources

The NHS Executive identified that 'the effective use of information management and technology is at the heart of the strategy to modernise the NHS'.* In order that this process is seamless, training has been identified as an essential requirement for a well-equipped workforce. PRIMIS (Primary Care Information Services) is an organisation that supports training in practices and PCOs to enhance the quality of data held on practice records.

PRIMIS has identified that:

- high quality data is needed to support NSF implementation, clinical governance and evidence-based practices
- comprehensive data aids call and recall systems and therefore clinical care
- data held are accurate and complete
- relevant and useful information needs to be extracted for a variety of clinical and non-clinical reasons
- PCOs will need to access information to support their commissioning role and monitor effectiveness of services
- data can be used to measure outcomes
- data facilitators improve the quality of information kept in the records, the dissemination of skills in the organisation and perform regular data extraction audits providing feedback for practices to focus on training issues.

---

* NHS Executive (1998) *Information for Health*. NHSE, London.

Further reading

NHS Executive (1998) *Information for Health*. NHSE, London.
NHS Information Authority (2002) *Caring for Information: a model for the future*,
    October. NHSIA, Birmingham.
PRIMIS facilitators handbook: http://www.primis.nhs.uk.

Access to records

A patient of yours for many years asks about accessing his medical records
held at the practice. His request comes 'out of the blue' during a routine
consultation. The patient makes it clear that he has no complaints about his
medical treatment but he is interested in seeing what has been written in
his notes over the years.

1   What 'rights' does the patient have regarding access to his notes?
2   Who can access the patient's records?
3   When should access be denied?
4   What are the implications to the practice in time, cost and manpower?

Patients' rights on access

There are two important acts of legislation that allow patients to access their
medical records. The first was the Access to Health Records Act 1990, which
allows patients to access any record in their notes made after 1 November 1991.
This resulted in notes made before this date still being out of the reach of the
public. A further law was passed which allowed access to notes in their entirety,
which we know as the Data Protection Act 1998, which came into force from
1 March 2000. This allows patients, or third parties acting on their behalf, entitle-
ment to access to their full medical records including manual and electronic. Prior
to both Acts patients had no rights to see any part of their records.

Who can access medical records?

There are a variety of circumstances when individuals can apply for access (*see*
individuals' rights in Chapter 2).

Parental consent
The Children's Act 1989 defines the rights and responsibilities of parents and who
fulfils these rights. Persons over the age of 16 years old are entitled to confidentiality in their own right. Best practice indicates that children under 16 years old
are encouraged to include their parents in decisions about their medical care.

From 1 December 2003, unmarried fathers will also be able to gain parental
responsibility by registering the birth of the baby together with the mother, from
this date. The other route will be to apply for a parental responsibility order
through a court order or a signed official agreement with the mother.

For electronic records, consultations are often conducted with the screen on full view to the patients. This informal sharing between the patient and doctor can be an aid both to improving communication, and a better understanding by the patient of what information is held on their record and if this information is correct. Conversely there may be times when a third party is present when confidentiality may prevail. This encourages the use of screen savers and passwords to prevent unauthorised access to notes.

A useful consent form for obtaining access can be found in the DoH *Guidance for Access to Health Records*.

Denial of access

There should only be a few circumstances when a request for access to records may be denied (*see* individuals' rights in Chapter 2).

Complaints on access

Patients who have a complaint regarding access to their medical records can either complain:

- to the individual health professional via the current practice complaints procedure
- through the NHS complaints procedure
- to the Information Commissioner, or
- seek legal redress.

Cost implications to the patient and the practice

Formal applications are made in writing to the practice, normally to the practice manager or the GP. The health professional responsible for the patient must then make a decision about disclosure, bearing in mind that there are only rare circumstances when information may be withheld. The practice may charge for access to the records. There are standard BMA fees for access and copies of records (*see* box).

	Access only	*Access and copies*
Manual notes	£10	Up to £50
Part manual/computer	£10	Up to £50
Electronic notes	£10	£10

The patient must be informed of the charges for access, and practices may charge 'reasonable' fees of up to £50 for access and copies, unless the records are computer/electronic-based, which incurs a lower fee. Any manual records added to within the last 40 days may be accessed free of charge. Patients should be given access within 21 days of the written request and appropriate fee. Requests may take up to 40 days; any delays likely to take longer than this should be communicated to the patient. Once access has been given to a patient, there is no obligation to give further access to the records until a 'reasonable' time interval has elapsed. Illegible notes must be interpreted and terminology explained to the patient. No charge can be made for this service by the practice irrespective of the time that may be needed.

Access

- Staff entering comments on patients' notes must remember that patients will have access to them.
- Prior to the legislation, the notes may contain comments that were never intended for patients to see.
- The BMA recommends that GPs discuss any 'potentially distressing entries' before showing them to the patient, which may be amended or deleted.
- Patients must have access before notes are amended.
- Access may be denied.
- Patients can have copies of notes and a fee may be charged.
- Records must be provided within 21 days.
- Explanations of terminology must be given.
- If patients require explanations of the notes, this must be provided.
- Access to the notes of deceased patients is not covered by the Data Protection Act but by the Access to Health Records 1990, which only applies to notes made after 1 November 1991.

Further reading

Data Protection Act 1998.
Children's Act 1989.
DoH (2003) *Confidentiality: NHS Code of Practice*, version 3.0. http://www.doh.
gov.uk/ipu/confiden
DoH (2003) *Guidance for Access to Health Records Requests under the Data Protection Act 1998*, version 2, June.

Patient consent to access medical information

The local PCT has a public health research fellow working with the commissioning group for local services. To accurately assess the local need for alcohol services, the research fellow would like to conduct an audit within the practice, collecting data on alcohol consumption in the local population. Although the data is anonymised the senior partner is unhappy with this sensitive information about the local population being used in this manner.

---

1   Why is patient information so essential for the NHS?

Use of patient information

Proposed changes to patient consent to release personal information are contained within the Health and Social Care Act 2001 (section 60). A consultation exercise is currently occurring which will look at proposals to allow for patient-identifiable information to be processed without the patient's consent. This change in the law will allow organisations to obtain patient-identifiable information for medical purposes, where it is impractical to gain consent from the patient. This will include information held on the following databases:

- NHS-wide clearing service
- hospital episode statistics
- national health authority information services
- patient episode data for Wales.

Information supplied to these databases is used in:

- commissioning healthcare services
- call and recall cancer services
- monitoring performance
- producing statistics on healthcare services essential for NHS activities and outcomes.

Consultation is currently taking place between the newly formed Patient Information Advisory Group (PIAG), parliament, the DoH and the wider community.
For further information on PIAG *see* www.advisorybodies.doh.gov.uk/piag

Complaints procedure

The practice manager regularly reviews the policies in the practice. As part of a rolling programme of continuing professional development for the practice, the practice complaints procedure is due for updating. The manager is keen to produce a simplified version for use by patient groups within the PCO and the patients registered with the practice.

1   Why should the practice complaints procedure be reviewed regularly?
2   What should the procedure include?

Changes to the NHS complaints procedure

Legislation is constantly changing, requiring policies and procedures to be reviewed regularly within the NHS to keep abreast of these changes. Continued public involvement and 'openness' are part of the changing culture of the NHS. Primary and secondary care need to adopt procedures that allow standardisation across the NHS regarding patient complaints and hence simplification.

The Health and Social Care Act 2001 will also introduce:

- an independent complaints support service for people who want to complain about the NHS
- new powers for local government to overview and scrutinise the NHS
- a duty on the NHS to involve and consult the communities it serves.

The NHS complaints procedure came into effect in 1996 and set out a framework on how complaints should be dealt with in the NHS encompassing primary and secondary care providers. The external contributors to the complaints system will include the National Clinical Assessment Authority and the National Safety Agency.

Complaints procedure

The new recommendations currently under review include the following stages.

Stage 1

Local resolution

- Uniform procedure across primary and secondary care with consistent timeframes.
- Dissemination of good practice and greater use of conciliation.
- National targets for managing the performance of staff handling complaints.
- Standardised administrative and financial support.
- Clear lines of responsibility.
- Staff handling complaints are properly trained.
- Quarterly reporting to trust board level.
- Having a named individual responsible for handling complaints.

Stage 2

Independent review

- Consistent criteria for convening Independent Review Panels.
- The possibility of a regional NHS body or new Independent Review Authority.
- 'Fast track' system for specific cases.
- Wide circulation of the panels' final report.
- New options of how panels should be convened.

The new system is intended to bring consistency across the NHS, provide timely resolution and involve the public to a greater degree. Monitoring the outcomes from the review panels and disseminating best practice are additional benefits for the patients and NHS staff.

The Health Services Commissioner (Ombudsman) will still be acting in an independent capacity to investigate complaints on clinical issues involving healthcare professionals.

Further reading

The National Health Service (Complaints) Regulations (2004) Statutory Instruments Consultation Draft Act of Parliament. www.rcgp.org.uk/rcgp/information/publications

Confidential waste

The practice has successfully become paper light over several years. All the mail coming into the practice relating to patients' records are scanned into the notes. The redundant paper is currently stored in date order in a filing cabinet but it is becoming clear to the partners that storage is becoming a problem.

A decision has to be taken over what to do with this increasing mountain of paper.

---

1 What is confidential waste?
2 How can practices incorporate paper-based information into the electronic record?
3 What arrangements should be made for the storage of confidential waste?

Definition of confidential waste

Confidential waste can be regarded as any material that holds information that can be used to identify an individual patient. If the information has been incorporated into the electronic patient record then this material is redundant. Examples would include:

- used prescriptions and prescription requests
- paper containing information in the form of letters, laboratory reports, x-ray reports scanned into the electronic patient record
- floppy disks
- CD-ROMs
- hard drives
- the current paper medical record of the patient
- faxes relating to patients, containing identifiable information
- correspondence from patients
- reports relating to patients, e.g. medical insurance forms.

Incorporating information into the electronic record

There are various clinical systems for practices to choose from. Paper documents in the form of correspondence from medical colleagues, patients, outside agencies and laboratory results are often scanned into the computer system for storage and incorporation into the patient's clinical record. Retention of medical records has previously been described which applies to both paper and electronic records.

Those practices relying on electronic storage of medical records have the additional burden of incorporating paper documentation into the electronic record, which can be retrieved in an accurate form. Information held in the paper form is often scanned into the system. There are two basic types of image recording. An optical reader scans the image into the system, but the scanned image must be checked, so that the image is a true copy of the original document. Checking must ensure no errors are transferred from the original document. The other type of scanner involves taking a photographic image and storing the document as an electronic photograph. Current recommendations are that paper records can be destroyed after scanning only if a facsimile of the original document can be produced and the practice has appropriate safeguards in the practice to prevent destruction of any part of a patient's medical record. This will include the practice having adequate backup procedures of copying information recorded during the day's work, use of backup tapes and storage of the tapes in a secure, off-site facility.

Storage of confidential waste

The practice will need to have regular and ongoing training for the PHCT to enable the information to be recorded correctly, stored safely and confidentiality maintained.

The storage of large amounts of paper records can become difficult for practices. It has always been the responsibility of practices to ensure records are held in secure facilities. It is also the responsibility of practices and PCOs to ensure that they have the capacity to store both paper and electronic records. Any additional storage of practice records becomes the responsibility of the PCOs in the interim years.

All paper documentation after the required length of storage needs to be destroyed as confidential waste. Any material in the practice with identifiable information relating to patients will also have to be treated as confidential waste.

Information being transferred from paper records into the electronic patient record should result in the paper records becoming confidential waste.

The medical defence organisations would advise practices to keep all records pertaining to any ongoing complaint or medico-legal case.

Summary

Confidential waste

- Any material that has patient details which could lead to a patient being identified.

- This includes letters, prescriptions, laboratory results, sick notes, insurance and disability forms.
- Shredding reduces the chances of material being identified.
- Commercial firms specialise in the treatment of confidential waste for general practice.
- Written material scanned into computer systems can be destroyed immediately if a facsimile of the original document can be produced in its entirety. Appropriate safeguards must be in place in the system to avoid loss of the medical record.
- PCOs hold the responsibility for storage of written records if practices run out of space.
- Remember that electronic records held on hard drives and floppy disk/ CD-ROMs constitute confidential material and organisations must take steps for information to be wiped prior to disposal of the computers.

Electronic records are covered by a comprehensive range of guidelines produced by the DoH, which covers the arrangements practices must make in order to become paperless. The guidance also covers assessing training needs of individuals using clinical systems in the practice, and consent from patients when using data from their notes.

Further reading

General Practitioners Committee/DoH (2003) *Good Practice Guidelines for General Practice Electronic Patient Records*, September. GPC/DoH.

Electronic communications

The office supervisor complains about a receptionist to the practice manager. The complaint revolves around the amount of time the receptionist is accessing the Internet. The receptionist claims the work is related to 'patient care'.

1   What areas need to be covered in an 'email and Internet use' policy in the practice?
2   What can the partners do as employers to monitor this situation?

Areas that need to be covered in the practice relating to email and Internet use

Electronic messaging in the form of internal and external emails and Internet usage is an increasing form of communications for healthcare in the modern NHS. The ability to access web pages containing information from recognised professional bodies, up-to-date medical information and various online evidence-based publications is an invaluable resource to the PCOs.

Patients as the wider public are an increasing group of Internet users for leisure and work purposes. Practices who are experienced with computerisation may offer their patients the opportunity to communicate with the practice via this media. This communication, while benefiting the patient, practice, administration staff, PHCT and doctors, also poses a variety of issues to consider.

Practice websites

PCO and practices may have the opportunity to have a website to promote the practice and include general information, services provided, personnel employed, and how to contact the practice. This may include information on the variety of methods of contacting the practice. Information may be found on a website for the practice or the PCO.

Practices may provide the opportunity for patients to email the practice directly to request prescriptions or to have a specific query answered. When responding to a patient's request it must not be assumed that the email reply will only be seen or accessed by the patient. Depending on the content of the email, it may be considered not appropriate to send via this route; consider a written communication or a face-to-face discussion with the patient. Simple acknowledgement of the request may be all that is required.

Internet access

NHS staff should currently have access to a wide range of information through the use of the Internet. This results in personnel requiring a range of computer skills to facilitate this access. Accessing this information and dissemination among individuals can vastly improve the level of knowledge among the PHCT on key issues, e.g. NICE guidelines, NSFs.

While access to web pages connected with work is totally appropriate, unfortunately Internet users may inadvertently find themselves connected to web pages that could be considered offensive or inappropriate. There should be in place a reporting system in the event of this occurring, for the protection of the Internet user. The importance of password log-ins, to prevent unauthorised use of computers and provide a clear audit trail, must be emphasised, to protect innocent individuals and also employers who may be asked to provide evidence for alleged breaches of indecency.

Practices should have in place adequate policies and procedures within the practice to guide staff in responding to and dealing with emails and Internet use.

Internal messaging

Emails are a common method for individuals to communicate within the practice and between practices, using conventional software packages. Many practices have the facility to incorporate separate software packages to enable them to use instant on-screen messages. This results in an increased accessibility of personnel to each other with resultant advantages and disadvantages. Usually there is a 'filter' available to screen out non-urgent messages at inappropriate times and to avoid interruption to the individual, e.g. if consulting with patients.

Any emails containing personal information that can identify a patient must be regarded as confidential, as with any other part of a patient's record.

With increasing use of instant messaging or emails within a surgery, a written record is generated. This may be a general enquiry asking for advice on a range of issues or with regard to a patient's disease, or information that should be shared across the PHCT about a patient. When details are entered that allow the receiver to identify an individual patient, then the correspondence can be considered as part of the patient's record. With the advent of the Freedom of Information Act, patients will be entitled to see the written records of emails kept regarding information of their condition or comments made about them.

External messaging

Emails can be an effective method of communicating quickly to colleagues and patients. This method of communicating can also increase the accessibility of individuals to each other. As NHS staff become more electronically competent, care must be taken to protect the confidentiality of the content of email, information relating to identifiable patients, and protection of the users themselves.

Practices will usually have anti-virus software in place to protect the computer system from corruption from intentional and unintentional virus infection. Often a common disclaimer is added to each external message.

Staff should be encouraged to respect patient details as confidential material and treat the information in a sensitive manner.

Monitoring electronic communications

Each individual should have a personal user name and password that is unique to that individual. Personal emails should be marked as such, and should remain confidential to the user. Under the Data Protection Act employees may still find themselves subject to a range of interventions at work including 'monitoring' of emails, which can be systematic, when an employer monitors all employees. 'Occasional' monitoring is an alternative process when an employer introduces monitoring in a short-term measure in response to a particular problem. Examples include:

- inappropriate or offensive material/content, e.g. text or images relating to ethnicity, race, disability, sex, sexual orientation, religious or political beliefs
- monitoring procedures by employers if excessive use during working hours
- suspected malpractice
- inappropriate downloading from websites, e.g. pornography.

Employers need to justify that any adverse impact on employees due to monitoring is justified by benefits to the employer. Employers need to discuss any monitoring procedures with the employees and obtain their consent. For 'interception' which results in recording of personal information an employer will need to satisfy both the Regulation of Investigatory Powers Act and the Lawful Business Practice Regulations 2000 and the requirements of the Data Protection Act. Consultation with trade unions is currently not mandatory under employment law but employers should ensure that processing the personal information is fair.

'Covert' monitoring would include measures that employees would not be aware of. It is only used in exceptional circumstances, e.g. when a criminal activity is suspected. Usually evidence needs to be collected within a certain timeframe. Once the investigation is complete the covert monitoring would cease.

Electronic communications would also include telephone, fax, voicemail and Internet access as well as email.

Emails

- Consider if emails are the most appropriate method of communicating sensitive information.
- Passwords should be used at all times both for the clinical records and for access to personal emails and Internet use. This will ensure a full audit trail.
- The practice should have a policy in place for the use of email and Internet access.
- Emails containing information identifying a patient must be treated as confidential and become part of the patient record. As such patients are entitled to have access to them (Data Protection Act).
- The content of emails within a practice may be subject to public access (Freedom of Information Act).
- Email records are of equal weight legally as written records and therefore due consideration should be applied.
- Do not assume replies to patient email enquiries will be treated confidentially as they would within the practice.

Further reading

Information Commissioner (2003) *The Employment Practices Data Protection Code. Part 3: Monitoring at work.*

Publication scheme

The practice manager returns from a PCO meeting and informs the partners that the practice needs to comply with new legislation regarding a 'publication scheme' allowing patients and the general public to access information regarding the practice details along with the current practice policies.

---

1   Why should information about the practice be released into the public arena?
2   What is the current legislation to enable this change to occur?
3   What types of information may the public and patients request?

The need for changes in the culture of information sharing

The general public perception of GPs, and the practice at which they are registered, is centred on the care they receive as patients and the services offered.

Most patients are not aware of the vast array of skills and personnel required to provide clinical care for patients, the administrative aspects, managing staff, audits, and maintaining links with PCOs and acute hospital trusts, to name a few.

General practices could be considered as being managed as a 'small firm'. For those GPs who retain independent practitioner status and employ staff directly, the GP retains responsibility for their employed staff. Salaried doctors are employed by the PCO and PMS doctors can either be employed by the PCO or retain independent status. Their staff may also have the option of employment with the PCO.

As such, partners not only conduct clinical meetings with staff, but often have to hold managerial meetings and long-term planning for the future running of the practice. The skills required to manage the administrative aspects of the practice effectively have grown over the years so that specific personnel have to be employed to bring in those skills. Practice managers need to handle aspects of accounts, cash flows, staff budgets, quarterly accounts, financial planning, formal complaints and disciplinary procedures. Partners often hold financial meetings or separate partners' meetings to discuss the strategic and financial running of the 'company'. Agendas and minutes of the meeting are usually held within the practice and are circulated to the appropriate members of staff.

As practices merge, there is a growing complexity and incorporation of business affairs into the primary care setting.

Some practices are so advanced that 'planning' days are held away from the practice, for key personnel to discuss the strategic business plan for the forthcoming year.

With the increasing investment in primary care, from public funds, we are often responsible for large amounts of public funds, especially so in a large practice. We therefore have a responsibility to ensure that this money is spent wisely and efficiently for the provision of patient services. Previously this information has remained within the domain of the practice and the PCO.

Legislation to enable sharing of information from general practices

The Freedom of Information Act (*see* Chapter 3) legislates that all NHS organisations, including GP practices, have a publication scheme to promote information being shared within a practice into the public domain. This will tell the public what information the organisation holds and will be publicised on either the practice or PCO website. Information also has to be made available to the public in paper form, for those who do not have access to the Internet. Practices may charge only for printing costs, which should be minimal and the cost to the public clearly shown.

Types of information the public may access

It is hoped that this introduction of legislation will provide the public with the necessary information about public services and promote accessibility and openness.

A selection of material may include:

- a range of practice policies, e.g.
  - complaints procedures
  - prescribing policies
  - confidentiality policy
  - a policy explaining why a patient may be removed from the practice
- staff employed at the practice
- how the practice is funded and resources allocated to the practice
- quality scores achieved from the new contract
- details of how the information is made public and any charges for accessing the information
- keeping information up to date.

An electronic version has been developed to help practices comply with the new legislation. *See*: www.foi.nhs.uk/redtape.

Exclusions:

- practice accounts
- information relating to national security
- law enforcement
- commercial interests
- personal information
- harmful information to the public
- harmful information to the commercial interest of a third party.

A variety of policies are to be found in Chapter 6, which will assist practices comply with the publication scheme. The policy provided can be adapted for local needs of the practice.

Significant event analysis

The practice is informed of the recent death of a patient by suicide. The PHCT decides to use this incident to review the practice's approach to patients with severe enduring mental illness. A significant event analysis is used to review the case. During the review several areas are found that require improvement and changes are made within the practice. Unfortunately the practice receives a complaint from the family who request all the relevant medical records are made available to their solicitor.

1 Why is significant event analysis useful?
2 What are the potential drawbacks of significant event analysis?

Use of significant event analysis

Significant event analysis or significant event auditing (SEA) is a technique that provides a structured approach to case discussions. SEA has been an important educational tool to aid individuals and teams improve the quality of care given to patients. Medical audit had been used in the secondary care setting since the 1970s, focusing on mortality rates. Applying this technique to primary care was first described in 1995 and has been refined to look at events that have occurred in day-to-day clinical practice, ranging from clinical near misses to administrative issues. Often the cases are discussed within a multidisciplinary team to provide a setting to maximise the full potential for change and improving clinical care.

There are a variety of templates available to record the events and outcomes.

There are many benefits to gain from SEA both for individuals and for the wider PHCT.

Significant event analysis

- An important learning tool.
- Benefits individuals and teams in providing improvements in care.
- Anonymous data can be used effectively to bring out learning points.
- Care should be taken when looking at contentious cases.
- Consider how records of the event will be stored and used in the future.
- The new GP contract awards quality indicators for significant event reviews.

Learning outcomes include:

- personal reflection on case study
- tackling teamwork issues and improving multidisciplinary working
- incorporating evidence from the literature into working practices
- improvements in quality care provided to patients
- reducing risks to patients and staff in future
- changes in practice protocol
- linking learning into practice development plans.

Potential pitfalls

SEAs, by their very nature and content, begin to look at controversial areas. The new contract suggests areas including complaints and aspects of patient care in which there has been a cancer diagnosed or death/suicide. While the team explores these issues there may be individuals or systems which have resulted in sub-optimal care. Although these issues can result in reflective learning for the learner, there will also be resultant changes for the individual/team in approaching care for patients in the future.

It must be remembered that if information is shared which allows the patient to be identified, then it must be regarded as confidential. In the event of any litigation regarding a patient's care, then discussion of that patient becomes part of the patient record. Care must be taken in recording clinical details, events and outcomes from SEA, as written notes may be regarded as medical evidence and requested by legal colleagues.

Further reading

Pietroni R (2001) *The Toolbox for Portfolio Development*. Radcliffe Medical Press, Oxford.

Pringle M (2000) Significant event auditing. *Scand J Health Care*. **18**: 200–2.

Pringle M, Bradley CP, Carmichael CN, Wallis H and Moore A (1995) *Significant Event Auditing: a study of the feasibility and potential of case-based auditing in primary medical care*. Occasional paper 70. RCGP, London.

Report to the Royal College of Physicians. *Medical Services Study: deaths under 50*.

Rughani A (2001) *The GP's Guide to Personal Development Plans*. Radcliffe Medical Press, Oxford.

The new GP contract

> The partner responsible for finance in the practice has spent several sessions reading the new contract and discussing with the practice manager the necessary changes that will be required.
>
> There are a range of issues that need to be incorporated into the practice to fulfil the requirements of the contract and gain the maximum quality indicator points.

1 What quality indicators can successfully be covered with the help of this text?
2 What statutory requirements can be achieved with the information provided in this text?

The new contract

New contractual agreements for GPs and their staff came into force from April 2004. There are several areas in which practices will aspire to achieve standards laid out in the new contract. A range of quality indicators within the contract are relevant to the previous information on confidentiality, access, record keeping and education. Chapter 6 on practice policy documents will also assist practices in achieving a high standard of care for the practice and primary healthcare staff. The policies will also act as a starting point for complying with the publication scheme and statutory requirements of the new contract. There is a range of legislation in progress to support the implementation of the new GP contract.

Quality indicators

Records and information about patients

Records 4 1 point	There is a reliable system to ensure that messages and requests for visits are recorded and that the appropriate doctor or team member receives and acts upon them.

See office policy for visits and messages in Chapter 6.

Records 14 3 points	The records, hospital letters and investigation reports are filed in date order or available electronically in date order.
Records 15 25 points	The practice has up-to-date clinical summaries in at least 60% of patient records.
Records 18 8 points	The practice has up-to-date clinical summaries in at least 80% of patient records.
Records 19 7 points	80% of newly registered patients have had their notes summarised within eight weeks of receipt by the practice.

See retention of records in this chapter.

Patient communications

Information 3 1 point	The practice has arrangements for patients to speak to GPs and nurses on the telephone during the working day.
Information 4 1 point	If a patient is removed from a practice's list, the practice provides an explanation of the reasons in writing to the patient and information on how to find a new practice, unless it is perceived such an action would result in a violent response from the patient.

See practice policies, removal of patients.

Education and training

Education 2 4 points	The practice has undertaken a minimum of six significant event reviews in the past three years.
Education 6 3 points	The practice conducts an annual review of patient complaints and suggestions to ascertain general learning points which are shared by the team.
Education 7 4 points	The practice has undertaken a minimum of 12 significant event reviews in the past three years, which include (if these have occurred): • any death occurring in the practice premises • two new cancer diagnoses • two deaths where terminal care has taken place at home • one patient complaint • one suicide • one section under the Mental Health Act.

See significant event analysis in this chapter; practice complaints policy in Chapter 6.

Practice management

Management 10 4 points	There is a written procedure manual that includes staff employment policies including equal opportunities, bullying and harassment, and sickness absence (including illegal drugs, alcohol and stress) to which staff have access.

See Chapter 6 for a variety of example policies.

Contractual and statutory requirements

Practice leaflet
The new GP contract also specifies that information has to be provided for patients regarding the opening times and services offered by the practice. The requirements to produce this information will be supported by legislation.

See practice leaflet in Chapter 6.

Complaints procedure
The practice has to inform patients on how complaints will be dealt with in the practice and that the practice policy complies with the NHS complaints procedure.

See practice complaints policy in Chapter 6.

Patient access to records

The practice has a system to allow patients access to their records on request with current legislation.

See access to records, p. 151.

Caldicott Guardian

There is a designated individual (data controller) responsible for confidentiality.

See Chapter 1, Section 1, Caldicott Guardian/information governance lead.

Electronic computer records

If the records are computerised there are mechanisms to ensure that the data are transferred when the patient leaves the practice.

See confidential waste, p. 156.

Data Protection Act

If the team uses a computer, it is registered under and conforms to the provisions of the Data Protection Act.

See Chapter 1, Section 1.

Electronic transmission of data

The practice has a written procedure for the electronic transmission of patient data which is in line with national policy.

See electronic communications (p. 158), safe havens (pp. 47–54), retention of records (pp. 52–3).

Further reading

BMA (2003) *New GMS Contract: investing in general practice.* BMA, London.

Further information

Websites

Publication scheme (online registration for practices)
www.foi.nhs.uk/redtape

Information Commissioner's Office
www.dataprotection.gov.uk

Department for Constitutional Affairs
www.lcd.gov.uk

British Medical Association
www.bma.org.uk

General Medical Council
www.gmc-uk.org

National Clinical Assessment Authority
www.ncaa.nhs.uk
020 7273 0855

National Patient Safety Agency
www.npsa.nhs.uk

Addresses

Security and Data Protection Programme
NHS Information
15 Frederick Road
Edgbaston
Birmingham B15 1JT
Tel 0121 625 2711
Fax 0121 625 1999

Information Commissioner's Office
Wycliffe House
Water Lane
Wilmslow
Cheshire SK9 5AF
Tel 01625 545700
Fax 01625 524510

British Medical Association
BMA House
Tavistock Square
London WC1H 9JP
Tel 020 7387 4499

General Medical Council
178 Great Portland Street
London W1W 5JE
Tel 020 7580 7642

Health Services Commissioner (Ombudsman)
England
11th Floor
Millbank Tower
Milbank
London SW1P 4QP
Tel 020 7217 4051

Wales
4th Floor Pearl Assurance House
Greyfriars Road
Cardiff CF1 3AG
Tel 01222 394621

Scotland
28 Thistle Street
Edinburgh EH2 1EN
Tel 0131 225 7465

Northern Ireland
Progressive House
33 Wellington Place
Belfast BT1 6HN
Tel 01232 233821

Freephone Health Information Services 0800 665544

Chapter 6

Practice policies

Introduction

This chapter looks at practice policies and some thoughts as to why policies may be beneficial to general practices, in the light of changes occurring in the new GP contract and evolving legislation. There are obvious practical advantages and considerations to take into account, as general practice continues to develop and strive towards providing a high standard of care to its patients and continually improving the services provided to those patients.

With the introduction of the publication scheme and the new contractual obligations in the new GP contract, practices will soon become aware of a variety of issues within general practice that will require clear written information for the general public to access.

Quality indicators

The new GP contract includes a variety of quality indicators linked to the various activities to be found within a practice. Details of specific indicators relating to Caldicott, data protection, confidentiality and access of records can be found in Chapter 5. Any material or templates that would facilitate the practice meeting those standards are also referenced in this chapter.

Contractual and statutory requirements

Also to be found in the new GP contract are specific requirements to comply with the introduction of the new GP contract. The standards set out in the new contract are to be adhered to if the contract is accepted by the practice. Although the areas are clearly defined and must be achieved, there are no additional points or financial reward attached. The main themes included in the new GP contract, for which relevant material may be found in this text, are:

- practice leaflets (standard 1)

    - an outline of the minimum requirements is on p. 178

- procedure for handling patients' complaints (standard 2)

    - *see* practice complaints procedure (pp. 179–85)

- Details of how patients can access their medical records (standard 11)

  – *see* access to medical records page (pp. 102–5)

- a named Caldicott Guardian (standard 12)

  – *see* Caldicott Guardian (pp. 10–11)

- Data Protection Act (standard 14)

  – *see* Caldicott manual (pp. 95–101)

- procedure for the electronic transmission of patient data (standard 15)

  – *see* safe havens (pp. 47–54 and 14–17)
  – *see* email and Internet policy (pp. 13–14).

The primary healthcare team

Practice policies are designed to help the practice, and the individuals who work there, work cohesively and effectively together. Designing a policy within a team allows everyone to contribute. The team agrees on a set of 'rules' around a policy area, a defined standard if relevant, which can be incorporated into the policy and the policy distributed throughout the staff for consultation and an intention to implement within a timeframe.

Policies are written with the intention that they are followed in a prescriptive way, unlike guidelines, which may be interpreted by individuals depending on circumstances. Response to policies may be varied. While some individuals may welcome the introduction of policies, others may find them restrictive and even oppressive to their natural way of working.

Advantages

- Defines a set of 'rules' that everyone can follow.
- Consistency in standards of care, e.g. diabetic clinic protocol.
- Risk reduction, e.g. rheumatoid blood monitoring policy.
- Improves teamwork.
- Transparency within a practice.
- Promotes a professional and organised approach to problems.
- Incorporates learning from internal review, e.g. auditing appointment availability.
- Incorporates learning from external review, e.g. legal requirements.
- Resolves differences of opinion within a team.

Not everyone will agree with the introduction of policies for a variety of reasons. Individuals can find standardisation and the perceived loss of individuality difficult to adjust to. Discussion with the whole PHCT prior to induction of a policy can overcome most of the initial fears and prejudices.

To reduce the amount of work a team may have to contribute towards writing a policy, outline templates are provided in this chapter.

Disadvantages

- Loss of individuality, e.g. prescribing policies.
- Policies may remain just an idea, unless disseminated and to a degree enforced.
- Source of conflict between team members when not adhered to.
- Policies can never cover all contingencies.
- Need for regular review and updating of policies to maintain and improve standards.
- Tendency to become outdated when compared against external reference, e.g. changes in legislation.

Publication scheme

The Freedom of Information Act legislates that all NHS organisations, including GP practices, have a publication scheme to promote information being shared within a practice into the public domain. This will tell the public what information the organisation holds. The practice is intended to inform the public in a variety of ways. Information also has to be made available to the public in paper form, for those individuals who do not have access to the internet. Practices may charge only for printing costs, which should be minimal and the cost to the public clearly shown.

Quality awards

There are several awards, which individuals and PHCTs may work towards, that are based around work-related issues. Often there will be a set criterion or standard which the individual and/or practice will have to show evidence of achieving.

Fellowship by Assessment and Quality Practice Awards, acquired from the Royal College of General Practitioners, have a variety of specific clinical and non-clinical areas requiring written evidence of policy adoption in general practice.

Incorporation of policies into general practice

Careful consideration must be given when introducing a policy into the practice. There are several areas within general practice that lend themselves well to the 'practice policy' concept.

- Administration

  - handling repeat prescription requests
  - house call requests
  - dealing with appointment requests
  - IT security and coding
  - office protocols.

- Employment:

  - staff contracts
  - disciplinary procedures
  - sickness and absence monitoring
  - harassment and bullying
  - grievance procedures.

- Legal requirements:

  - access to records
  - data protection
  - health and safety
  - confidentiality.

- Clinical governance:

  - national service frameworks
  - external national and local standards
  - complaints procedure
  - Caldicott requirements.

- Clinical areas:

  - prescribing policies/practice formulary
  - chronic disease management
  - drug monitoring.

Essential components of a policy

As with any document a series of essential 'core' sections are often a framework, around which the themes and ideals of a policy are built. There will always be a need for additional sections to be added for specific issues relating to an individual policy. Local adaptation is an aspect that allows practices to incorporate key aspects of a policy relating to their work, allowing for practical challenges and local needs to be incorporated.

The core elements could include the following.

Basic core elements

- Justify why the policy is needed.
- Set out general principles.
- Define content or 'rules' to be followed.
- Who needs to follow the policy.
- Indicate how the policy will be implemented.
- Identify how the policy will be monitored.
- Clarify outcomes if policy not implemented.
- Set a timeframe for regular update and review of policy.
- Where the policies will be kept.

- How individuals will access them.
- Who will update policies.
- How new policies will be disseminated among relevant individuals.

Dissemination of policies

Once the practice decides to develop a new policy the PHCT must agree on a basic set of 'rules' which they will follow. A document is produced and given to individuals either in paper format or electronically as email. It is usual to allow a period of consultation for members of the team to feed back any concerns or modifications of the policy.

It may be useful to compare your draft policy with other practices that may be using a similar idea, for additional improvements. PCOs can be a good resource of a variety of policies and procedures that could undergo adaptation for local practice.

If there is general agreement a circulation list should include everyone who will use this new policy. Regular checks should ensure new members are added to the circulation list.

The practice has to decide on where the policy will be kept so staff can refer to the documentation if needed. It may be useful to incorporate all the practice policies within a central file, which could be a paper record kept in a convenient place, e.g. reception, so everyone can access the material easily. Alternatively, a copy can be kept on the computer system, which people could access as required. Additional copies can be printed off when required.

Monitoring the effectiveness of policies

Various triggers can cause policies to be drawn up. The need may occur from a significant event analysis, an audit, a complaint, a desire to harmonise prescribing, standardise administrative tasks, or promote teamwork, to name a few. Once a policy is circulated, how will the team know that implementation has occurred within the relevant areas of work?

The ability to show that a policy has brought improvements within practice has enormous benefits. The ability to demonstrate to staff the advantages gained is good for the staff, the doctors and the patients. The effects of change and improvement within a practice can be thought of in terms of outcomes.

- Audits are often used to look at data, to demonstrate improvements in how a system or process works, e.g. auditing the number of security breaches on an annual basis may show that training in Caldicott has resulted in improvements in levels of maintaining confidentiality.
- Monitoring complaints may highlight areas requiring improvements, e.g. a large number of complaints about the length of time for a routine appointment may lead to the adoption of a partial booking or advanced access system for patient appointments. Monitoring of complaints may also be used to reveal where improvements already occurred, e.g. all written complaints may be acknowledged within two working days.
- External standards include the RCGP (Royal College of General Practitioners) Quality Practice Award and Fellowship by Assessment, e.g. direct comparison

on how the practice complaints procedure compares with expectations from an external reference can provide focus on how the policy should be improved.

- Morale is often 'sensed' rather than measured by those who work together in a team. It is a very common issue for the primary care team, who are constantly striving to deliver high quality care to the public, often with limited resources.
- Efficiency could be measured in raw data, e.g. an increase in numbers of patients seen in a working week. Efficiency may need to incorporate more complex issues, e.g. patients who were seen by the most appropriate healthcare professional to suit their medical needs. This may result in an overall reduction in numbers of patients seen by a doctor in the surgery.
- Appraisals can often be a vehicle for staff to discuss aspects of their work which require further training or may provide the employer with an insight into the limitations of processes functioning within a practice. For example, a receptionist may ask for training on issuing repeat prescriptions but the underlying problem may be the methods of how patients request repeat medications.
- Clinical governance has always been and continues to be an important aspect of examining the standards of care we provide to patients. It allows the incorporation of 'best practice' into our clinical models, and assesses the performance of the PHCT in providing care to patients and providing a framework that links our work with education, training and continual professional development.

Changes in policy

Ultimately the practice policies will need to undergo regular review. This is essential to ensure that policies are changed in accordance with new legislation, changes in work practice, as a consequence of monitoring the effectiveness of a policy and as external standards become accepted and integrated in our day-to-day work.

A nominated individual, e.g. practice manager, may be best placed to ensure regular review is undertaken on each of the practice policies. Updated policies will need to be circulated and old copies destroyed to prevent confusion.

Summary

The rest of the chapter contains a variety of basic templates that could be found as a working policy within a general practice surgery.

The templates are designed to cover the basic themes currently under review in general practice and to assist practices to start redesigning their approach of sharing knowledge and information held within a surgery with the full PHCT and the wider public.

Templates are given in printed text, which can simply be photocopied and disseminated among the staff for consultation or use within the surgery.

The full text is also found on www.radcliffe-oxford.com/informationgov in Word or pdf format so that modifications can be made to the outline of the policy to incorporate specific needs of a particular practice or local working conditions. Once the template has been changed to satisfy the needs of the people who will be using the policy on a daily basis, then the modified document can be printed off for use.

General practice surgery details may be substituted in the appropriate blanks and the documents printed off for use by the practice, or disseminated electronically to those individuals who will be using them.

It is recommended that the practice check with the appropriate organisation – i.e. BMA, MDU, PCO – for advice prior to adoption of a policy, due to the changing legislation.

There are also a variety of 'templates' which can be accessed from commercial websites but often attract a fee.

Remember that the templates provided are a starting point for the practice to start reviewing what processes are currently used, whether all individuals are aware of agreed processes and how they can be improved to enhance the services delivered to the patients. An additional benefit could include risk management, as potential areas of concern may be highlighted before an incident or complaint occurs.

The following templates are provided

- practice leaflet
- practice complaints policy
- office policy.

Further reading

1   RCGP quality standards.
2   New GMS Contract 2003.

Practice leaflet

Practice leaflets are a useful and simple way of providing patients with information about the surgery and the services provided by the PHCT. Practice leaflets can be updated on the computer and printed off as required or accessed via the practice website if available. Practice leaflets have been an essential requirement for training practices and for GPs undergoing Fellowship by Assessment at the RCGP.

New patients attending for registration may find the information within the leaflet particularly useful, to familiarise themselves with the range of services provided by their new practice.

Under the publication scheme practices may wish to provide information in the practice leaflet on how to obtain access to the full range of policies used within the practice.

The style and format of the practice leaflet may have various forms, as there are no set requirements apart from the content. Practices may prefer to use a printing firm to produce a professional looking booklet. Cost and constant changes to the content of the practice leaflet may inhibit some practices in using these types of services. There are a wide variety of software packages for computer users to enable them to produce and design a document incorporating the requirements of the 'practice leaflet'. This method has the advantage that regular changes within the surgery can be easily incorporated into the practice leaflet and disseminated to the patients. PCOs may have personnel who can assist practices with training requirements for this type of skill. *See* www.opg.co.uk.

This list forms the basis of the contractual and statutory requirements for a practice leaflet as stated in the new GP contract from April 2004.

Practice Leaflet

[Name of Practice]

[Address]

[Telephone number]

[email]

- Practice opening hours.
- Whether an appointment system is used.
- The appointments times for doctors or nurses.
- How to access a doctor or nurse.
- Services provided by all members of the practice team.
- How patients can access these services.
- How to obtain repeat prescriptions.
- How to make a complaint or comment on the services provided.
- Patients' rights and responsibilities.
- How the practice uses personal health information.

[insert name of practice]

Practice complaints policy

Introduction

[Name of practice] is committed to ensuring that all patients receive the highest standards of care. From time to time, patients or the patients' representative may wish to complain about an aspect of their care. It is in the interests of the practice and patients that complaints are dealt with promptly and with a degree of sensitivity.

Types of procedure

Practice route

Most complaints are of a simple nature, informal, verbal, and can often be clarified by front-line reception staff in the course of their daily duties.

If, due to the nature of the complaint, it will require more than a simple explanation, the complaint is passed onto an appropriate senior colleague, usually the practice manager. Details can be entered onto a complaints form if received verbally. The patient or their representative can also write to the practice directly. Consent from the patient must be obtained if a representative is acting on behalf of a patient.

Acknowledgement of the complaint will occur within two working days. The complaint will be investigated and a written reply should take place within 20 working days. In usual circumstances, when it may not be possible to reply by this timescale (e.g. an absent staff member), then the complainant will be written to, with an expected date for a reply.

When a complaint involves a clinical issue, any healthcare professional involved should also receive a copy of the complaint, as soon as it is received by the practice. It is the responsibility of the healthcare professional to discuss the complaint with their defence organisation, if appropriate.

Most complaints can be answered by writing to the patient with an explanation of what has occurred, what changes have resulted from the complaint, and/or an apology. If the complaint is resolved a copy of all correspondence should be kept for future reference.

If patients are not happy with the outcome of the complaint, they may seek an alternative route.

PCO route

The person for dealing with any complaints in our practice is [insert named person].

The person dealing with complaints in the PCO is [insert name].

The practice will endeavour to work with the PCO to resolve your complaint as quickly as possible.

In the initial stages of a complaint the PCO may offer the services of a conciliator (*see* box) who will meet with the practice and the complainant to cover the areas of the complaint. The conciliator will listen to both sides and try to deal with any outstanding issues from either side to try to resolve the complaint. The conciliator is not there to make a decision or judgement on the complaint.

The conciliator

- An independent lay person.
- Usually skilled in dealing with complaints from patients.
- Undergoes regular training to help parties resolve a complaint.
- Experienced listener and facilitator.
- Selected on their level of skill.
- Usually selected from a list developed through the strategic health authority.

This process may involve the practice representatives and the complainant meeting separately with the conciliator. The option for the complainant and practice representatives to meet together at a later stage is always available during the resolution of a complaint.

Independent review of complaint

If resolution of the complaint has not been achieved the complainant can ask for an independent review of the complaint by the PCO. This is a panel formed by the PCO. The panel is asked to look at the issues involved in a complaint. The panel usually consists of:

- one or two independent lay persons chosen from a list held at the local strategic health authority
- lay chairperson
- clinical assessors, which are typically one or two GP specialists or possibly a consultant involved in the relevant medical field associated with the complaint
- complaints convenor, usually a lay person from the PCO or strategic health authority.

The group will consider the complaint, view all relevant correspondence and clinical records, listen to all individuals involved, ask relevant questions and then give recommendations. The possible outcomes include:

- refer to the General Medical Council, informing the PCO clinical subgroup and chief executive
- refer the complaint back to the practice for further resolution if the panel feels inadequate local resolution has not taken place
- dismiss the complaint
- written recommendations to the practice following full investigation of the complaint – the PCO may be required to provide ongoing support and involvement in the practice depending on the recommendations of the panel.

Independent routes
General Medical Council
At any stage in a complaint the public may complain directly to the GMC. The GMC is an independent body and can be contacted on Tel: 020 7580 7642 or in writing at 178 Great Portland Street, London, W1W 5JE or via www.gmc-uk.org.

Legal redress

Patients may seek advice from a solicitor regarding an aspect of their medical care. Relatives may also seek advice on behalf of the patient. Often the patient or relative may seek access to the medical record so a third party (legal representative) can advise the complainant.

Ombudsman

The Ombudsman or Health Services Commissioner is an independent body with the authority to investigate clinical complaints and complaints about healthcare professionals.

If the complainant is not satisfied with the NHS complaints procedure, including the independent review, they must write to the Ombudsman within a year of the complaint coming to light. All supportive written information needs to be included, which would also involve material from the independent review. The complainant must state why they are not happy with the independent review.

The decision the ombudsman makes is final; there is no appeal.

Monitoring

For effective monitoring of this policy, complaints requiring a written reply, copies of the complaint, reply and final resolution will be kept at the practice for future reference.

Complaints that involve the PCO will also be monitored through the PCO clinical governance process.

Review of procedure

This policy may be amended at any stage through consultation.

Confidentiality

All aspects of a complaint, either verbal or written, will be treated as strictly confidential.

Members of staff, who may be involved with the complaint, may not discuss the details of the case outside the practice. Breach of confidentiality may lead to disciplinary action.

Proposed changes

The GMC are currently working towards a single 'gateway' for complaints for healthcare professionals and NHS care. The Healthcare Commission are proposing a phone line, website and information leaflets to help patients determine which route they wish to take regarding a complaint.

There are also changes outlined in *Reforming the NHS Complaints Procedure* which may mean that patients may complain directly to the PCO without informing the practice, which is currently the usual route. The proposals would also give the Healthcare Commission responsibility for independent review panels, which would result in no clinical involvement with the complaint panel.

Further reading

DoH (2001) *Reforming the NHS Complaints Procedure: a listening document*, September.

[PRACTICE NAME]

[PRACTICE ADDRESS]

[PRACTICE TELEPHONE NUMBER]

[PRACTICE WEBSITE]

Office policy

[DATE]

Contents

- Practice statement.
- Confidentiality.
- Mail.
- Messages.
- Visit requests.
- Prescriptions.
- Visitors.
- Practice complaints procedure.

Practice statement

[Name of practice] is committed to ensuring that all patients receive the highest standards of care possible, from the medical, nursing and administrative staff. It is expected that patients are treated in a courteous and sensitive manner.

We endorse a non-discriminatory and non-ageist policy. We will endeavour to try to provide services for those patients with special needs, i.e. disability, language difficulties, ethnic/cultural requirements.

As a practice we encourage suggestions from patients and staff, which will improve our services and standards of care.

We operate a zero tolerance policy towards verbal and physical abuse of staff, in accordance with the latest NHS policy. Patients exhibiting such behaviour will be instantly removed from the practice list.

Confidentiality

- All staff must to be aware that the information held in the surgery is confidential. This applies to a patient's medical records, either in electronic or paper format. It also includes any additional information that relates to a patient's

personal circumstances. Any data that includes information that can identify a patient must be regarded as confidential.
- This same level of confidentiality also applies to other NHS staff responsible for patient care.
- Any concerns or queries should be discussed with the Caldicott Guardian [insert name of Guardian for practice] here at the practice.
- Staff will be required to read the full policy in the practice's schedule.
- Training on all aspects of confidentiality will be provided, and requires ongoing regular updating.

Mail

- All mail is opened and stamped with the date.
- Items are distributed between the doctors who are in the practice that week. Mail should go to the doctor identified by name.
  If doctors are absent (i.e. holiday and sickness) for any given week, their mail will be distributed to the remaining doctors for vetting and appropriate action.
- All items of mail (including laboratory results, letters, investigation results) should be dealt with by the nominated doctor. Non-urgent mail would include items such as insurance forms and disability living allowance forms, which may be left until the relevant doctor dealing with the patient has returned from leave.
- Urgent faxes or reports should be given to the addressee on the fax. In their absence the fax will be shown to the nominated doctor available at the time for a decision or action.

ALL INFORMATION VIEWED IS STRICTLY CONFIDENTIAL.

Messages

- Messages are directed to a nominated member of staff on a daily basis.
- Messages are [written down in the message book] [recorded in electronic format] as they are received
- Non-urgent messages can be left until the end of surgery.
- Recipients will [sign the message book] [have a record in electronic format] to indicate they have received the message.
- Patients are reminded to ring [insert times of day] for results in accordance with details set out in the practice leaflet.
- Emergency requests or messages should be dealt with as quickly as possible. The relevant doctor should be contacted within [time limit] to be informed of the request. If members of staff are not clear of the degree of urgency, they should consult a senior colleague for advice.

Visit requests

- A nominated member of office staff is responsible for visit requests during working hours.

- Requests for home visits can be either by letter or telephone – *see* practice leaflet.
- Patients are requested to ring [times] on the day for a non-urgent, same-day visit.
- Non-urgent requests for house calls are logged in the [visit book] [electronic format]. A contact number, address, patient details and if possible a brief description of the 'problem' should be recorded. Patients may request a specific doctor.
- Under certain circumstances, it may be necessary to interrupt the doctor, while in surgery, when it is apparent from the nature of the telephone request that the patient is seriously ill. If in doubt, please seek advice from an experienced member of staff. Training will be provided to enhance your telephone skills. When no doctor is available on the premises, a doctor will be able to be contacted by [mobile telephone] [bleep].
- House call requests are usually divided up between the doctors who are available that morning. The practice must have a mechanism in place, which clearly indicates to the member of staff which doctors are available for house calls.
- Requests for visits after [time] must be passed on to the doctor on-call via the usual contact method. The details of the house visit are recorded in the usual manner. The staff must be aware which doctor is responsible for visits at certain times of the day when requests for visits are logged.

Prescriptions

- Patients may request their prescriptions by telephone, letter or email.
- Most requests will be dealt with within two working days.
- A notice in reception will advise the patient when their prescription will be ready for collection, if the request arrives before [time] on the day.
- A nominated member of staff will deal with repeat prescriptions, which include drugs that a patient receives on a long-term basis. Such medication will be recorded in the patient's notes. This medication will be authorised by the doctor, to be printed on a prescription by administrative staff, and then be checked and signed by the doctor. Staff will receive specific training for this duty.
- If the medication cannot be found in the appropriate system or the drug needs authorising by the doctor, then the system will not allow the staff to print the prescription. In those circumstances, the request is passed onto the doctor.
- A clear system for repeat prescribing must be in place so that a responsible doctor is identified to deal with the prescription request. There is an audit tool for repeat prescribing in the Appendix.

The doctors operate a surveillance policy to ensure patients on repeat medications are reviewed on a regular basis.

Visitors

- [Name of practice] has a variety of visitors on a daily basis.
- A clear notice in the reception area asks visitors to report to the reception desk. Visitors may include those who have appointments with clinical or administrative staff.

- *All* visitors should be dealt with courteously. Please inform the relevant person of their arrival.
- A visitor's book at reception is an essential part of our health and safety policy. Please ask visitors to fill in their details, and remind them to sign the book on their departure.
- Unknown visitors are not allowed to wander around the building unaccompanied.

Practice complaints procedure

- [Name of practice] is committed to ensuring that all patients receive the highest standards of care. From time to time, patients or their relatives may wish to complain about an aspect of their care. It is in the interests of the practice and patients that complaints are dealt with promptly and with a degree of sensitivity.
- Patients who wish to complain, but show excessive verbal or physical aggression, should be referred to the office supervisor or practice manager if available.
- For a full description of the practice complaints procedure, please consult the full practice policy schedule.

Appendix

Prescribing incentive scheme
Repeat prescribing model audit 1

Aim of the audit

To review your current repeat prescribing system and identify areas for improvement. Criteria to be audited include:

- Presence of directions on prescriptions.
- Equivalence in terms of number of days treatment to be supplied.

Sample size

The sample size for the audit is to be proportional to your practice list size. You will need to review the medical records for x number of patients where x **is equivalent to 2% of your practice list size**. For example, if you have a practice list size of 6000, you will need to include 120 patients in your repeat prescribing audit.

Method

Use the data collection sheet supplied for collecting the data. This you will need to photocopy as many times as necessary.

1 Determine the sample size for your audit as explained above.
2 Decide when you are going to commence the audit and inform your reception staff.
3 From the commencement of the audit period, reception staff should note down consecutively the **names of patients** for whom repeat prescriptions are requested and **their date of birth or computer number**. (This is so you will be able to identify the patient when you come to examine their medical notes and/or repeat prescription record).
4 Staff should continue to note down patient names until enough have been recorded for your sample size, e.g. 120 patients for the example given above.
5 Note down the number of prescription items on the repeat prescription record for each patient.
6 Note the number of 'active' prescription items on the repeat prescription record that **lack directions** for the patient or state 'as directed'.

7   For multiple items on the repeat prescription record, record if the quantities stated are **equivalent in terms of the length of supply**, e.g. all 28 days, all 30 days or all 56 days. 'When required' prescriptions and prescriptions for original packs are excluded. (If you utilise the 'number of days treatment' box on the prescription form, ensure that this is always for the same period of time and that directions are given for each prescription.)

Analysis of results

Calculate:

a   The proportion (%) of items on the repeat prescription record that have directions for the patient, excluding items where directions are not applicable, e.g. 'non-active' items such as dressings and stoma products and insulins and anticoagulants:

% items that have directions

$$= \frac{(\text{total number of items} - \text{number of items without directions})}{\text{total number of items}} \times 100$$

b   Where applicable, the proportion (%) of repeat prescription records where the number of days to be supplied is equivalent:

% repeat prescription records, where applicable, that are equivalent

$$= \frac{\text{number of repeat prescription records that are equivalent}}{(\text{number of equivalent records} + \text{number of inequivalent records})} \times 100$$

Standards

Now you have examined your current performance in repeat prescribing you need to set standards for the level of performance you would ideally wish to achieve. Below are given some **examples** of standards.

Criteria	Standard (example)	Standard (set your own)	Date undertaken .... Your actual achievement:
Where applicable, all items on repeat to have directions for the patient (excluding specified exceptions defined by the practice clinician(s) prior to the audit)	80%		
Where applicable, multiple items on a repeat prescription to be equivalent in terms of length of supply			

Implement change

The repeat prescribing system audit will have identified areas relating to repeat prescribing where you have achieved your desired standard and others where you have not.

For those areas where you did not perform as well as you may have liked, you will need to implement a change to your repeat prescribing system in order to improve your performance.

If you **did** achieve your desired standard, was that because the standard was set too low?

Re-audit

Once you have implemented the necessary changes to your repeat prescribing system, a re-audit should be carried out.

Incentive scheme

A summarised report of the audit and how effective the changes introduced as a result have been, should be received by the PCT no later than 31 March.

Model Audit 1 – Data Collection Sheet

Patient identifier (Practice number)	Patients' Date of Birth	Number of items on Repeat Prescription Record	Number of 'Active' items without directions or state as directed	Equivalent (number of days supply) Yes, No or Not applicable (N/A)

Prescribing incentive scheme
Repeat prescribing model audit 2

Aim of the audit

To review your current repeat prescribing system and identify areas for improvement. Criteria to be audited include:

• Presence of discontinued/redundant prescription items on the repeat prescription record.
• Equivalence in terms of number of days treatment to be supplied.

Sample size

The sample size for the audit is to be proportional to your practice list size. You will need to review the medical records for x number of patients where **x is equivalent to 2% of your practice list size**. For example, if you have a practice list size of 6000, you will need to include 120 patients in your repeat prescribing audit.

Method

Use the data collection sheet supplied for collecting the data. This you will need to photocopy as many times as necessary.

1 Determine the sample size for your audit as explained above.
2 Decide when you are going to commence the audit and inform your reception staff.
3 From the commencement of the audit period, reception staff should note down consecutively the **names of patients** for whom repeat prescriptions are requested and **their date of birth or computer number**. (This is so you will be able to identify the patient when you come to examine their medical notes and/or repeat prescription record.)
4 Staff should continue to note down patient names until enough have been recorded for your sample size, e.g. 120 patients for the example given above.
5 Note down the number of prescription items on the repeat prescription record for each patient.
6 Note the number of prescription items on the repeat prescription record that have not been requested in the last six months.
7 For multiple items on the repeat prescription record, record if the quantities stated are **equivalent in terms of the length of supply**, e.g. all 28 days, all 30 days or all 56 days. 'When required' prescriptions and prescriptions for original packs are excluded. (If you utilise the 'number of days treatment' box on the prescription form, ensure that this is always for the same period of time and that directions are given for each prescription.)

Analysis of results

Calculate:

a The proportion of prescription items on the repeat prescription record that are current, i.e. have been requested in the last six months:

% items on the repeat prescription record that are current

$$= \frac{\text{total number of items on repeat prescription record} - \text{total number of items not requested in last 6 months}}{\text{total number of items on repeat}} \times 100$$

b Where applicable, the proportion (%) of repeat prescription records where the number of days to be supplied is equivalent:

% repeat prescription records, where applicable, that are equivalent

$$= \frac{\text{number of repeat prescription records that are equivalent}}{\text{number of equivalent records} + \text{number of inequivalent records}} \times 100$$

Standards

Now you have examined your current performance in repeat prescribing you need to set standards for the level of performance you would ideally wish to achieve. Below are given some **examples** of standards.

Criteria	Standard (example)	Standard (set your own)	Date undertaken .... Your actual achievement:
Prescription items on the repeat prescription record to be current (requested within the last six months) (excluding specified exceptions determined by the practice clinician(s) prior to the audit)	90%		
Where applicable, multiple items on a repeat prescription to be equivalent in terms of length of supply	80%		

Implement change

The repeat prescribing system audit will have identified areas relating to repeat prescribing where you have achieved your desired standard and others where you have not.

For those areas where you did not perform as well as you may have liked, you will need to implement a change to your repeat prescribing system in order to improve your performance.

If you **did** achieve your desired standard, was that because the standard was set too low?

Re-audit

Once you have implemented the necessary changes to your repeat prescribing system, a re-audit should be carried out.

Incentive scheme

A summarised report of the audit, with those items excluded from the six-month repeat rule, and how effective the changes introduced as a result have been, should be received by the PCT no later than 31 March.

Model Audit 2 – Data Collection Sheet

Patient identifier (Practice number)	Patients' Date of Birth	Number of items on Repeat Prescription Record	Number of items on Repeat Prescription Record that have not been requested in last six months	Equivalent (number of days supply) Yes, No or Not applicable (N/A)

Further reading

Anderson RJ (1996) *Security in Clinical Information Systems*, January. Consultation paper commissioned for the BMA Council by the BMA Information Technology Committee.

BS 7799-1:1999: *Information Security Management Part – 1: Code of practice for information security management.* http://www.nhsia.nhs.uk/erdip/pages/docs_egif/evaluation/technical/ehr-req-final.pdf

Data Protection Act 1998: http://www.hmso.gov.uk/acts/acts1998/19980029.htm.

The Data Protection Act 1998: an introduction: http://www.dataprotection.gov.uk.

DoH (1997) *The Caldicott Committee Report on the Review of Patient-identifiable Information*, December. http://www.doh.gov.uk/ipu/confiden/app2.htm

DoH (2003) *Confidentiality: NHS Code of Practice*, version 3.0. http://www.doh.gov.uk/ipu/confiden

EL(92)60: *Handling Confidential Patient Information in Contracting: a code of practice* (issued 1992).

GMC (2004) *Confidentiality: protecting and providing information.* The GMC provides detailed guidance on consent on its website: http://www.gmc-uk.org/standards/.

Guide to the Practical Implementation of the Data Protection Act 1998 (DISC PD 0012 1999) http://www.bsi.org.uk/pd12

HSC 1998/64: *The Management of Health, Safety and Welfare Issues for NHS Staff* (issued April 1998).

HSC 1998/217: *Guidance for GP Medical Records (Retention Periods of Records).*

HSC 1999/012 outlines the person specification and role of the Guardian.

HSC 1999/053: *For the Record: managing records in NHS trusts and health authorities.*

HSC 2000/09: *Protection and Use of Patient Information.*

HSG(96)18: *The Protection and Use of Patient Information* (issued March 1996).

IG Toolkit: http://nww.nhsia.nhs.uk/infogov/igt/RequirementsList.

Information Commissioner (2002) *Use and Disclosure of Health Data: guidance on the application of the Data Protection Act 1998*, May. http://www.informationcommissioner.gov.uk

NHS Executive (1996) *Guidance on Video Recording NHS Operations*, issued under cover of a letter from the Chief Executive.

Published by the Confidentiality Issues Section of the NHS Executive: *Protecting and Using Patient Information: a manual for Caldicott Guardians* (issued March 1999) http://www.doh.gov.uk/confiden/index.htm.

Published by the NHS Executive's Security and Data Protection Programme and available from the NHS Information Authority:

- *Ensuring Security and Confidentiality in NHS Organisations* (E5498) 1999.
- *The Handbook of Information Security: information security in general practice.*
- *Play IT Safe: a practical guide to IT security for everyone working in general practice*, version 1.1, 1999.

NHS Information Authority Code of Connection.

NHS Information Authority Security and Access Policy.

NHSnet Code of Connection.

PRIMIS facilitator's handbook: http://www.primis.nhs.uk/.

The NHS, DoH, BMA and the clinical professions have agreed that patient identifiable information should be encrypted before being disclosed via any external network. *See* encryption and cryptography section of http://www.nhsia.nhs.uk/confidentiality/pages/standards.asp.

Glossary

Access control	It ensures the use of a resource by an authorised person and also includes the prevention of use of a resource in an unauthorised manner.
Anonymised information	It is any information or combination of information which does not identify an individual directly, and which cannot reasonably be used to determine identity.
Authorisation	The granting of rights, which includes the granting of access based on access rights.
Availability	Information is disclosed to the authorised person, when needed and in a usable form.
Backup	The process of taking copies of data and software with the intention of being able to restore them if they are damaged in any way.
Commissioner	Is an independent officer who is appointed by Her Majesty the Queen and whose duties are specified in Chapter 7 of the Data Protection Act 1998 and who also supports the enforcement of the Freedom of Information Act.
Confidentiality	Data access is confined to those with specified authority to have access to that data.
CRAMM	The CCTA Risk Analysis and Management Method.
Data controller	A person (or persons) who determines the purpose for which and the manner in which personal data are, or are to be, processed.
Data owner	An individual having responsibility for a specified logical or physical set of data and for the maintenance of appropriate security measures.
Data subject	An individual who is the subject of personal data.
Disclosure	The divulging or provision of access to data.
Encryption	Information in plain-text format is converted into characters and codes using privacy-enhancing technology so that it cannot be understood if intercepted in transit. The recipient decodes it.

Explicit or expressed consent	Interchangeable terms meaning an articulated agreement, given orally or in writing, as a clear and voluntary indication of a preference or choice.
Health professional	A person who is a registered: medical practitioner, nurse, midwife, health visitor, osteopath, chiropractor, dentist, optician, pharmaceutical chemist or a clinical psychologist, child psychotherapist or speech therapist.
Health record	Any record which consists of information relating to the physical or mental health or condition of an individual, and has been made by or on behalf of a health professional in connection with the care of that individual.
Identification	The method of an individual stating his/her identity to the Information Technology system.
Impact	Comprises embarrassment, harm, financial loss, legal or other damage which could occur in consequence of a particular security breach.
Implied consent	A patient's agreement that has been signalled by behaviour of an informed patient.
Information security	Protection of information to ensure its confidentiality, integrity and availability.
Integrity	All components of the systems are operating correctly according to specification and in a way the current user believes them to be operating.
Log-in, log-on	The procedure whereby a user obtains admittance to the IT system, establishing his/her identity at the same time.
Log-off, log-out	The procedure whereby a user leaves the IT system.
Maintenance	The upkeep of computer equipment and/or software.
NHSnet	A NHS-wide network that allows universal transfer of messages, subject to the requirements of security. The goal is for any NHS organisation to be able to exchange information with any other, securely, cost-effectively and irrespective of the hardware or software supplier.
Password	Confidential authentication information composed of a sequence of characters. The password should be known only to the individual concerned.
Patient	In this book the term 'patient' is defined broadly and is also used synonymously for client and service user.
Patient-identifiable information	Any information which directly or indirectly may identify a person, for example: patient's name, initials, sex, address, full postcode, date of birth or death, NHS number, national insurance number,

local patient-identifiable codes, pictures, photographs, videos, audio-tapes, religion, ethnic group, occupation and such like.

Primary care organisation	Umbrella term for organisations involved in commissioning including primary care trusts and primary care groups.
Primary care trust	Organisation that commissions services on behalf of its constituent practices. Primary care trusts also commission community and social services.
Primary healthcare team	The clinicians or healthcare professionals in a general practice or associated with that practice, together with the administration team (practice manager, receptionist, secretary).
Processing of data	Processing means (in accordance with the Data Protection Act) obtaining, recording or holding the information or data, or carrying out any operation or set of operations on the information or data.
Public interest	In order to serve a legitimate societal interest in exceptional circumstances it justifies the overruling of the right of an individual to confidentiality.
Restore	Means obtaining the backed-up data or software and moving them into the operational directories ready for use.
Risk assessment	Concept for assessing the potential impact of threats to, and vulnerabilities of, computer systems, data and materials and capabilities, and for optimising investment in security countermeasures.
Safe-haven procedures	An agreed set of administrative and physical security procedures for ensuring the safe and secure handling of confidential patient information including guidance on the handling of records.
Security breach	Any event that has, or could have, resulted in loss or damage to NHS data and/or material, or an action that constitutes a violation of NHS security procedures.
Security policy	A statement of the set of rules, measures and procedures that determine the physical, procedural and logical security controls imposed on the management, distribution and protection of confidential sets of data and/or materials.
Sensitive personal data	They are ethnic origin or race, religion, mental or physical health, sexual health, political opinion, trade union membership, court proceedings or findings, conviction for an offence.

Sensitivity	A measure of importance assigned to information to denote its confidentiality.
Software	A generic term used for computer programs of all sorts, which includes the operating systems, application programs, utility programs or any other programs.
Third party	An identifiable person within a set of information who is
	• not the data subject
	• not the data controller or
	• any data processor or other person authorised to process data for the data controller or processor.
Threat	An action or event which might jeopardise security.
Virus	A self-reproducing program loaded without the knowledge of the user. Frequently viruses are harmless for a while, after which they will deliver their 'payload' and may destroy data and software.
Vulnerability	A security weakness.

Index

Page locators in *italics* refer to figures.

Access to Health Records Act (1990) 102, 123
access to patient records 102–5, 151–3
  applicant rights 102, 151
  correcting mistakes 105
  costs and charges 152–3
  deceased person's records 103–4, *153*
  parental access 102, 151–2
  protocols and procedures 102–3, *104*, 121
  staff corrections *153*
  timetables 153
  withholding disclosure 103, 121–2, 152
agencies and contract staff, confidentiality
    undertakings 33, 35, *36–7, 38,* 139
answering machines 14
appraisals and annual reviews (staff) 134
archived material 156–8
  outsourcing storage 53
  storage security 49, 53
  see also confidential waste
automated decision-making systems 100

backing-up data 59, 146
  storage 48
bank staff *see* agencies and contract staff
BS 7799 national standard for security 57

Caldicott Guardians 6, 45
  and IM&T security 63
  person specifications 10
  register of data 'owners' *46*
  responsibilities and roles 10–11, 63
Caldicott Principles 8, 133, 137
  case scenarios 129–46
Caldicott Report 5–7
  recommendations 5–6
CCTV use
  accountability 11
  disclosure policy document *109*
  protocols and codes of practice 13, 60–1,
    106–7, *110*
  recording retention period 49
  replay and application forms *111–14*
  security policy document *108*
change management 172–4

assessment of proposals 172–3
incorporation considerations 173–4
insuring relevancy 174–5
policy dissemination 175
evaluating effectiveness 175–6
updating and reviewing 176
child protection, information disclosure 124
Children's Act 1989 124
coded identifiers 6, 9, 139
codes of conduct for staff 12–13, 132–3
  office protocols 182–5
common law duty of confidentiality 117
communication with patients 30, 122–3,
    130–1, 161–3, 167
  basic principles 26–7
  legal requirements and obligations 26,
    27–8, *166,* 177–8
  new GP contract requirements *166,* 177–8
  patient information leaflets 27–8, *28–30,*
    177, *178*
  websites 159
  see also telephone use
complaints procedures 154–6, 167, 179–81
  informing patients 181–2
  office protocols 185
computer equipment security 58–9
  disposal policies 60
  identification and inventories 58, 143
  insurance claims 143–4
  maintenance tasks 59–60
  repairs and service contracts 59
  virus protection 59
  see also computer systems security policies
Computer Misuse Act 1990 78, 123
computer software
  automated decision-making systems 100
  copyrights 123–4
  vetting procedures 59, 76
  virus protection 144–6
computer systems security policies 57–61
  backing-up data 59
  Caldicott Guardian/information lead's
    role 63
  legal position 78

computer systems security policies (*continued*)
  monitoring and auditing use   73, 74, 141–2
  preventing unauthorised use   49, 78–80, 141
  restricting physical access   78, 143–4
  third-party access   80
  use of games/other software   59, 76
  user registration procedures   78–80, 140–2
  user responsibilities   63, 76–7, 141, 142
  virus protection   59, 144–6
confidential waste   156–8
  definition   156
  disposal   13, 53–4, 60
  electronic records   148, 157
  guidance documents   4–5
  shredding documents   13, 53, 60
  storage   53, 100, 157–8
Confidentiality: NHS Code of Practice (DoH)   4, 5
confidentiality
  breaches by staff *131*, 134–5
  policy communication   26–31, 182–5
  signed undertakings   33, 35, *36–7*, 134–5, 139
  staff induction procedures   21–2, 132–3
  staff training programmes   24, 25, 132–4
  workplace precautions and guidelines   13, 133–4, 182–5
  see also Data Protection Act (1998); disclosure; legislative framework
'consent' (data processing)   97–8, 131, 153–4
  concepts and definitions   97–8
  disclosure without patient knowledge   24, 27, 99, 130–1, 154
  implied   98
  patient information needs   26–7
  sharing anonymised data   118–19, 130–1
contract staff *see* agencies and contract staff
Copyright, Designs and Patents Act 1988   123–4
CRAMM (CCTA Risk Analysis and Management Method)   65, 197
Crime and Disorder Act 1998   118–19

data corruption   146
data disposal arrangements *see* confidential waste
data 'ownership'   45, 136–7
  see also Caldicott Guardians
data processing
  principles of good practice   26–7, 96–100
  see also 'consent' (data processing); patient records
Data Protection Act (1998)   95–101, *95*
  first principle   22, 26, 96–8
  second principle   98–9
  third principle   99
  fourth principle   52, 99–100
  fifth principle   100
  sixth principle   100
  seventh principle   100–1

  eighth principle   101
  and individuals' rights   102–5
data protection notifications   11, 97
data quality   27, 50–2, 149–51
  accuracy   99–100
  benefits of electronic records   150
  ensuring relevancy   99
  general principles   51–2
  guidance documents   150–1
  staff training   149–50
  see also patient records
data storage   49, 53, 100
  retention periods   52, 100, 147–9, 157
  theft or losses   54
  see also archived material; safe-haven procedures
database restructuring   6
destruction of personal data *see* confidential waste
disclosure
  legal framework   18, 24, 97, 117–24
  patient consent   96–9, 119–20, 131, 153–4
  implied consent   98
  informing patients   119–20
  police information requests   118–19, 124
  public interest   118–19, 124, 154
  requests to withhold disclosure   12
  sharing anonymised data   118–19, 130–1
  sharing patient-identifiable data   154
  staff guidance and training   *18–19*, 24, *25*
  without 'consent'   24, 27, 99, 119, 124
  see also access to patient records; confidentiality; inadvertent disclosure

email use   158–61
  codes of conduct   13–14
  external messaging   160
  monitoring and security procedures   49, 145–6, 160–1
  virus protection strategies   144–6
  see also computer systems security policies
encryption   6, 197
Ensuring Security and Confidentiality in NHS Organisations (NHS Executive)   4

fax machines   14–15, 137–40
  cover sheets   *17*
  guidance and protocols   15–16, 137, 138
  safe-haven procedures   48, 138–40, *138*
floppy discs, disposal arrangements   60
FoI *see* Freedom of Information Act (2000)
FoI leads   120–1
For the Record (HSC 1999/012)   4
Freedom of Information Act (2000)   120–3
  accountability and responsibilities   120–3
  'publication schemes'   122–3, 162

General Medical Council, complaints procedures   180, 181

GP contract 165–8
  effects on practice 172–85
  implementation issues and management
    172–7
  new procedures and requirements 171–2
GP practices
  office policies and procedures 182–5
  practice statements 182
  'publications schemes' 30, 122–3, 130–1,
    161–3, 167, 177–8, *178*
  quality awards 173
  quality indicators 166, 171
  websites 159
  see also GP contract

The Handbook of Information Security (NHS
  Executive) 4
hard drives, disposal arrangements 60
Health and Social Care Act 2001 (Section 60)
  119–20, 155
house calls 183–4
The Human Rights Act 1998 117–18

illegible records, patient access 153
IM&T suppliers, patient privacy safeguards 6
IM&T training 141–2
implied consent 98, 198
inadvertent disclosure 134–5
incident reporting *see* security incidents
information disclosure *see* disclosure
information flows 4, 5
  Caldicott Principles 8
  organisation responsibilities 5–6
  review requirements 39
  review procedures 39–40
  review questionnaires *41–4*
Information Governance Lead *see* Caldicott
  Guardians
information governance strategies
  guidance and policy documents 4, 83
  implementation recommendations 91–2
  management accountability 6, 10–11
  overview of legislative framework 3
  patient feedback 31
  performance audit questionnaire *84–90*
  performance review tasks 92–3
Information Security Management Part 1
  (BS 7799) 4
information security policies
  general overview 57–8
  risk assessment and management 65–8
  staff responsibilities 76–7
  see also computer systems security policies;
    confidentiality; disclosure
information sharing
  anonymised data 118–19, 130–1
  child protection measures 124
  legal basis 118–24, 136
  patient-identifiable data 154

protocols 55, 136
transferring out of UK 101
see also disclosure
information transfers *see* disclosure; email use;
  information flows; information sharing
insurance claims, lost or stolen
  equipment 143–4
Internet safeguards 13–14, 159, 160
  see also email use

legislative frameworks 3, 95–124
  common law duty of confidentiality 3, 117
  computer use 78
  information sharing 118–24, 136
  information security 57
  see also individual statutes
litigation 181
log-on and log-off procedures 80, 141–2,
  198

mail *see* postal deliveries (incoming/outgoing)
maternity records, retention period 52
mental health records, retention period 52
messages 183

new GP contract *see* GP contract
NHS Code of Connection 14
NHS patient-identification numbers 6, 9, 139

ombudsman complaints procedures 181

paediatric records
  patient/parent access 102, 151–2
  retention period 52
password security 13, 79–80, 123, 140–1, *140*
  logging on/off 80, 140–1
patient choice 26
Patient Information Advisory Groups (PIAGs)
  119–20
patient information needs
  excluded materials *163*
  PHCT publications 30, 122–3, 130–1,
    161–3
  range of practice policies *163*
  see also communication with patients
patient records
  definition 50, 148
  disposal and destruction methods 13, 53,
    148
  guidelines for best practice 50–2
  handling principles 50
  new GP contract requirements *166*
  patient access 102–5, 151–3
  deceased person's records 103–4, *153*
  quality issues 27, 50–2, 99–100, 149–51
  rectifying mistakes 105
  retention periods 52, 100, 147–9, 157
  sharing anonymised data 118–19, 130–1
  sharing patient-identifiable data 154

patient records (*continued*)
    staff alterations   123, *153*
    staff training   149–50
    storage arrangements   49, 53, 156–8
    taken 'off premises'   53
    theft or losses   54
    tracking systems   52
    use of information   24, 27, 99, 118–19,
         130–1, 154
patient-identification numbers   6, 9, 139
pigeon holes   48
police information requests   118–19, 124
policy implementation *see* change management
postal deliveries (incoming/outgoing)   183
    safe-haven procedures   47–8
posters, for policy communications   30, 122–3,
     130–1, 162–3
prescription security   140–1, *140*, 184
Preservation, Retention and Destruction of GP
     General Medical Services Records (HSC
     1998/217)   4, 52
PRIMIS (Primary Care Information Services)
     150
prisoner health records, retention period   52
Protecting and Using Patient Information, a manual
     for Caldicott Guardians (DoH)   39–40
The Protection and Use of Patient Information
     (DoH)   5
Public Interest Disclosure Act 1998   124
'publication scheme'   30, 122–3, 130–1,
     161–3, 173

quality awards   173
quality indicators   166, 171

reception areas
    breaches of confidentiality   *131*, 134–5
    visitor protocols   184–5
    see also safe-haven procedures
Reforming the NHS Complaints Procedure (DoH)
     181
retention of records   52–3, 147–9
    electronic record deletion   148, 157
    guidance documents   4–5, 100
risk assessment and management   65, 199

safe-haven procedures   47–9, 138–40, 199
    defined   47
    fax machines   48, 138–40, *138*
    guidance document   22, 23r
scanning data *156*
Security in Clinical Information Systems (BMA)
     5
security incidents
    classification/types   69
    follow-up responsibilities   70
    monitoring arrangements   16, 70–2, 138
    staff reporting responsibilities   16, 70–2
    theft and damage   *142*, 143–4
shredding documents   13, 53, 60
significant event analysis   163–5
software protocols *see* computer software;
     computer systems security policies
staff codes of conduct   12–13, 132–3
    office protocols   182–5
staff contracts   33–4
staff induction procedures   21–2, 132–4
staff training   132–4
    aggression management   130
    confidentiality and disclosure issues   24, 25
    IM&T   141–2
    new GP contract requirements   *167*
    patient records entry practices   149–50
    significant event analysis   163–5

telephone use
    answering machines   14
    general safeguards   13
    messages   183
    safe-haven procedures   48–9
temporary staff, confidentiality undertakings
     33, 35, *36–7, 38*, 139
termination of employment, contract terms   33
tracking systems, patient records   53

virus checkers   145

waste *see* confidential waste
websites, construction and maintenance   159
withholding information   103, 121–2, 152
    at patient's request   12